the Veterinary Receptionist's HANDBOOK

2nd Edition

M. T. McClister, DVM, and Amy Midgley

Veterinary Medicine Publishing Group
A Medical Economics Company

Published by Advanstar Veterinary Healthcare Communications
8033 Flint, Lenexa, Kansas 66214.

Printed in the United States of America

Library of Congress Catalog Card Number 95-61831
ISBN 0-935078-56-8

10 9 8 7 6 5 4 3 2
First printing: August 2000

TABLE OF CONTENTS

		Page
Introduction		iv
Chapter 1	Making a Good First Impression	1
Chapter 2	Getting Organized	15
Chapter 3	General Administrative Policies	27
Chapter 4	Answering Clients' Questions	37
Chapter 5	Fee and Payment Policies	45
Chapter 6	Scheduling Appointments	61
Chapter 7	Handling Emergencies	79
Chapter 8	Interacting With Clients	95
Chapter 9	Your Role in Marketing	111
Chapter 10	The Importance of Diagnostic Tests	123
Chapter 11	The Importance of Vaccinations	129
Chapter 12	The Importance of Internal Parasite Control	139
Chapter 13	The Importance of External Parasite Control	151
Chapter 14	Dispensing Drugs and Supplies	157
Chapter 15	Common Surgical Procedures	167
Chapter 16	Common Medical Problems	177
Chapter 17	Commonly Asked Questions: Small Animals	191
Chapter 18	Commonly Asked Questions: Horses	217
	Appendices	
	Glossary of Veterinary Medical Terms	230
	Vital Statistics	257
	Index	258

INTRODUCTION

Congratulations! Being a receptionist in a veterinary practice is one of the most interesting and rewarding jobs you will ever have—and one of the most important positions at your veterinary clinic.

You represent the animal hospital. The doctor speaks through you. You are the first person clients meet when they come to the clinic and the last person they see when they leave. The impression that clients form about you is the one they will carry along of your clinic. In fact, statistics show that one of the main reasons why clients switch from one practice to another is that they've encountered an indifferent and unwelcoming attitude in the front office.

You are the welcoming committee, the pleasant voice on the telephone, the helpful hand in the reception area, the appointment secretary, the bookkeeper, the question answerer, the scheduler, the director of sales, and the public relations department.

You are a very important person!

The Veterinary Receptionist's Handbook is designed to help you in your job, whether it's your first day or you've got years of experience.

As you read this book, you will learn how to make clients feel welcome and how to demonstrate the care that your hospital provides their pets (your most important job!), how to be a good communicator (your other most important job!), and how to organize the many details of everyday life in a busy animal hospital (yes, your *other* most important job!).

If you're a new receptionist, you'll probably find it helpful to start with Chapter 1 and go through each chapter in order. Of course, any chapter may be referred to as needed for help with a particular situation. Or, if you're an experienced receptionist, you may want to customize the information to fit your clinic's policies and then keep the book within easy reach to be used as a reference.

You'll probably find that it's a good idea to tab some of the pages for quick reference. As you'll see, many of the pages contain information specific to your clinic, and you'll want to refer to them daily.

Every receptionist needs to be able to answer clients' basic questions. The more you understand everyday medical procedures, the less often you'll have to interrupt the doctor with questions. That's why Chapters 10 through 16 provide you with essential information on immunizations, surgery, parasites, and diagnostic tests.

Chapters 17 and 18, Commonly Asked Questions, list the questions clients most often ask veterinary receptionists about their pets. The appropriate answers—along with additional space to fill in more specific information about your clinic's services and policies—are included. The more you study these questions and answers, the more confident you will feel and the better you will be able to communicate the right information to your clients.

And you'll hear lots of new terms. So there's a glossary of common veterinary terms and abbreviations in the back of the book. Again, the more you study and commit these to memory, the more confident you'll feel and the more successful you'll be!

Best of luck in your career as a veterinary receptionist. There's no question that when clients see your smiling face, they'll know they've brought their beloved pets to the right place!

CHAPTER

1

Making a Good First Impression

How many times have you walked into a business and found yourself ignored by the people who work there? It's not a pleasant feeling, is it? It makes you feel angry or like turning right around and walking out. In fact, you didn't have a very good first impression of that business, did you?

The Receptionist's Golden Rule

You are the first person clients talk to on the phone and meet when they enter the waiting room. The image you project will give them their first impression of your hospital.

Your job as veterinary receptionist is to make sure your clients never feel ignored and to make each client understand how much you, the doctor, and the entire hospital staff sincerely care about his or her pet.

In fact, your golden rule is:

Make the clients feel welcome. Show how much you care that they've chosen your clinic.

When clients walk into your clinic, smile. Greet them, thier pets, and their children by name. If you are on the phone when clients walk in, smile and wave to let them know you have seen them and will soon be able to help them.

☛ TIP

Your clients like to know who you are, too. Wear a name tag that gives your name and title, or place a nameplate on your desk.

If you're new and don't know the clients, don't despair. If you're on the appointment system, you should know who will be coming in. If you're not on the appointment system, a sign-in sheet can be a valuable aid. If you have no idea who a client is, ask! Then smile and use his or her name. Introduce yourself, too!

◆ SAMPLE SITUATION

A client with no appointment walks in and asks to start the series of vaccinations on his new puppy.

You say: *"We will be happy to take care of that for you. What is your name?"*

Client: *"John Jones, and this is Tippy."*

You: *"Mr. Jones, I know this is Tippy's first visit, but have you been in with other pets?"*

Client: *"About two months ago I brought my cat in."*

You pull his chart and say: *"Yes, I see that on your chart. How is Felix feeling now? It will take me just a few minutes to set up a file on Tippy."*

You proceed to get all the vital information on Tippy, set up his file, then say: *"The doctor will see you and Tippy now, Mr. Jones. When you leave we'll set up an appointment for your next visit. That way we won't keep you waiting so long!"*

With this approach, you let the client know that he should make an appointment for a visit without scolding him for not having one that day.

In every situation, make sure clients see how glad you are that they have come to your clinic. If you do this, you automatically project a friendly, caring image of your clinic and help clients feel at ease and receptive as they head to the exam room to see the doctor. Remember, if a client receives an unpleasant welcome at your hospital, he or she can visit any number of other clinics.

☛ TIP

Act professional—that's what you are! There's no need to gush over a client and a pet. A smile, a pleasant tone of voice, and genuine interest in the client and pet are all that's needed.

The Five-Minute Rule

As friendly as you are, clients don't come to your clinic to spend time with you! They come to bring their pets to the doctor. So, another important rule you'll want to follow is:

Don't keep the client waiting.

Ideally, a client should not have to wait more than five minutes before taking his or her pet to an exam room. Circumstances (such as emergencies) occasionally will disrupt smooth traffic flow, but you'll find that the five-minute rule will help you—especially on days when the waiting room is full.

Use your five minutes with the client wisely. Verify the address and phone number to ensure your records are up-to-date. Be sure to ask the reason for the visit if this was not done when the appointment was made. (See Chapter 6.)

➤ POINT TO PONDER

All pets are created equal, especially in the eyes of the owner. A dog with a fancy pedigree is not "better" than a Heinz 57 mix. The qualities of a good pet—companionship, friendliness, and loyalty—cannot be put down on a registration form.

The Unavoidable Delay

There will always be times when a client shows up right on time for an appointment and the doctor is unavailable to see the pet. Lengthy surgical procedures, emergencies, or simply a long series of appointments can all throw your schedule off.

When this happens, explain the situation to clients, tell them how long a delay to expect, and give them the options of waiting or leaving their pets at the clinic and picking them up when it's convenient. You can also ask if they'd like to reschedule their appointments.

Most clients will choose to wait, so don't forget they're in the waiting room! Keep them posted on the doctor's progress and let them know about any changes that could make the wait longer or shorter.

◆ SAMPLE SITUATION

An injured dog has been brought to your clinic, and the doctor must stabilize it before seeing any more clients. When Mrs. Smith appears promptly at 10 a.m. for Mitzi's appointment, you smile and say:

"Good morning, Mrs. Smith. You and Mitzi are right on time, but we are running a little bit behind. The doctor had to stop to treat an injured dog, and I expect the delay to be about 20 minutes. I'm sorry for the inconvenience to you, and if you're unable to wait, I'll be glad to reschedule your appointment or keep Mitzi here for treatment until you can come back for her."

☛ TIP

When the schedule becomes disrupted, try to call clients in advance to reschedule. They'll appreciate the consideration, and you won't have impatient clients in the waiting room.

The Telephone: The Clinic's Lifeline

The waiting room is full. A dog is barking. A client's new kitten is halfway up the curtains. And, of course, the telephone is ringing. Wait! Don't touch that phone. Take a deep breath. Smile. *Now* pick up the phone and answer it.

The telephone is the clinic's lifeline. Without it, business would fade away. That's why it's so important to answer it properly. Your ability to project a good image of your clinic over the telephone depends on your being able to answer questions confidently and accurately (see Chapter 2) and on following your golden rule: Make the clients feel welcome and show that you care about them and their pets! This applies to *all* clients—those on the phone as well as those in the waiting room.

The first step when you answer the phone is to smile and use a pleasant tone of voice. Remember, *how* you say something can be more important than *what* you say! In fact, the most important parts of a telephone conversation are tone and inflection.

☛ TIP

The phone shouldn't ring more than twice before you answer it. If you can't answer it by the second ring, ask someone to answer it for you.

Next, identify your clinic and give your name. For example: "Main Street Animal Clinic. This is Debbie speaking." People like to know to whom they are speaking. It puts them at ease.

☛ TIP

When you are on the telephone, speak slowly and clearly. You are your clinic's communication link to the outside world. Be sure the outside world can understand you!

Step number three, believe it or not, is the hardest: Listen to what the person on the phone says. Let callers know you are interested in them and their pets.

➤ POINT TO PONDER

No client's question is too trivial, even if you have already answered it 10 times that day. When Mrs. Jones asks it at 6 p.m., it will be the first time for her. Treat her with the same courtesy and respect you gave the first client at 8 a.m.

The Hold Button

There will be times when you must put callers on hold while you research answers to their questions or finish some business with clients in the waiting room. Use your hold button as seldom as possible, but if you must use it, say, for example, "I am on the other line. May I ask you to hold for just a moment? Thank you." Get back to the caller as soon as possible and say, "Thank you for holding. How may I help you?" or "Thank you for holding. I have the information you wanted."

☛ TIP

Always give callers the option of having you call them back if they don't want to hold. Take the caller's name and number and confirm that someone will be there in five or 10 minutes to receive your call.

"I Need to Talk to the Doctor"

You will quickly realize that doctors are very busy people. The fewer times they are interrupted, the more time they have for medical work. Properly handled, routine calls need not interrupt their work.

But sometimes, no matter the question or situation, clients feel that they can get the right information only by talking to the doctor. These clients do not mean to belittle you. They simply do not know that anyone but the doctor is capable of answering their questions. When a client insists on speaking to the doctor, be cheerful and cooperative. Explain that the doctor is unable to come to the phone right now but that he or she will return the client's call at a certain time.

☛ TIP

Be sure to convey to the caller that the doctor is busy seeing patients, making rounds, or in conference—that he or she is busy doing something and not just "too busy" to talk to the caller.

Your clinic may want to set aside 20 to 30 minutes in the morning and the afternoon for the doctor to return phone calls. Then you can tell the client about what time to expect the call.

Emergencies, of course, are handled immediately. (See Chapter 7.)

➤ POINT TO PONDER

Clients pay for their time with doctors and they deserve their undivided attention. Don't interrupt patient visits with nonemergency questions.

Clinic Callback Policies

"How Is My Pet Doing?"

Anxious owners usually want to check on their hospitalized pets early in the morning, but the doctor may not have had a chance to make rounds when they call. Many clinics set a time for clients to call to check on hospitalized pets—for example, after 10 a.m. This gives the doctor time to check on hospitalized cases and postsurgical cases and to let you know about each pet's condition. Be sure to update reports on all animals by the designated time so you can give information promptly to callers. This reassures worried owners—and makes your job easier!

☛ TIP

A client's first concern when calling your clinic will be for the pet's condition. The next question will usually be, "How much is my bill?" Be sure you can answer both questions, especially for pets that will be discharged that day.

Anxious owners often will call earlier than the designated time. To put your clients at ease, it is best to know whether there has been a drastic change in their pets' condition. If not, reassure them and tell them you will have complete details shortly. Do not put clients off by saying, "It's too early for you to call." After all, you care about their pets as much as they do, so communicate your concern in a reassuring way.

Clinic Policy on Reporting Hospitalized Cases and Follow-up Phone Calls

◆ SAMPLE SITUATION

A client calls first thing in the morning and says, "I brought my dog in last night at 11 o'clock. He was hit by a car. How's he doing?"

First, verify that the pet is not in immediate danger. Then tell the client, "Bowser is resting comfortably this morning. The doctor will have the complete details of his case a little later this morning. May we call you back at that time to let you know more?"

Write a note to remind yourself or the doctor to call the client back. It's your job to be sure the call is returned.

Remember, the telephone works both ways. One of the best ways to project the positive, caring attitude of your clinic and to show your concern for your clients' pets is to follow up with your clients. Call the owners of all surgical cases the day after surgery and say, "This is Debbie at Main Street Animal Clinic. Dr. Smith wanted to know how Tippy feels today."

If time permits, follow up with the owners of ill pets as well. When owners are worried about their pets, nothing is as comforting as a call from a concerned veterinarian.

Your computer will help you keep track of follow-up phone calls. Enter recheck dates for all ill pets and surgical cases, and the names and phone numbers will appear on a recheck report on the appropriate date. If you don't have a computer, designate a space on each day's appointment schedule where you will write down the names and numbers of clients to be called.

The Hard-to-Understand Caller

Occasionally it will be hard to understand someone over the phone because he or she speaks indistinctly, has an accent or a speech impediment, or simply because of a poor connection. Maintain your pleasant tone of voice—don't lose your patience!—and admit that you are having trouble understanding him or her. Ask the caller to speak slowly and to spell out his name and phone number.

☛ TIP

When in doubt, SMILE! It is almost impossible to speak in an unpleasant tone of voice if you are smiling.

SUMMARY OF IMPORTANT POINTS

- Always ask the caller's permission to place him or her on hold.

- Always give the caller the option of being called back.

- Don't interrupt the doctor during an office visit for answers to routine questions.

Notes

CHAPTER

2

Getting Organized

"This is Mrs. Brown. I'm calling to check on Spot's lab work."

"This is Mr. Smith. How is Buster feeling this morning?"

"I'm Ms. Lake, and I just got a bill in the mail from you for $25, but I paid that last Thursday. Would you check on it for me?"

"This is Mr. Jones calling. Is Fifi's appointment scheduled for 10 a.m. or 10:30 a.m.?"

How Am I Going to Keep Track of All This?

What You Should Know	How You Should Organize
1. How to give clients information that will help answer questions.	1. Until you know the answers, knowing where to find the answers is the next best thing.
2. Your clinic's policies.	2. Read your clinic policy manual, and keep it handy for quick reference.
3. Your clinic's procedures.	3. As time permits, observe the doctor during procedures and treatments. It will be much easier to explain the spay operation to a client if you understand it.
4. Details of everyday clinic business.	4. Set up a system of notebooks and calendar reminders to help you keep track of all those important details.

The four client questions listed on the previous page are only a few examples of those that you will be asked every day in your job as a veterinary receptionist. You've probably been asked at least some of them already.

In order to project a confident, caring image of your clinic, *you* must appear confident—not flustered. The best way to appear confident is to *be* confident, and confidence comes with knowledge and organization.

☛ TIP

Don't be afraid to tell clients that you don't have answers to their questions. Research the questions and report back to clients with the correct information. It is much better to say, "I don't know, but I'll be happy to find the answer for you" than to give clients incorrect information.

Now let's take a look at each of the organizational tips in our chart in greater detail.

Know Where to Find Information

Starting a new job is like moving to a new town. You can't find your way around during the first week or so without a map. Your first week on the job should be devoted to familiarizing yourself with your surroundings.

• Are appointments kept in the computer or in an appointment book? How are appointments scheduled?

• Where are your accounts receivable—the list of people who owe the clinic money? Are they tracked using a computer, or are they kept manually?

• Where is your list of fees and services?

• Where is your hospital's policy manual?

• Where are the client and patient files?

• Where are the forms for lab work—both to send lab work out and to take reports by phone?

• Where are the files for hospitalized patients kept?

• Where are the surgical files kept?

• Where are the files for patients who are ready to be released from the hospital?

• Does your clinic keep a daily status sheet on hospitalized cases? If so, where is it kept?

Spend your first few days on the job making a "map" of your clinic. By the end of your first week, you will have at your fingertips most of the essential information you need to do your job confidently and professionally.

☛ TIP

Remember, if you've never worked for a veterinary practice, you're going to be bombarded with lots of new information. Don't try to memorize everything at once. Instead, focus on learning where you can go to find the correct answers.

Understand Your Clinic's Procedures

Procedures govern the day-to-day operation of the clinic. For example:

• Does your hospital use an appointment system?

• Are appointments scheduled throughout the day or only between certain hours? At what times does the doctor return phone calls?

• Does the client have to pay at the time of the visit, or will the next week be okay?

• What days is the clinic open? What are the clinic's business hours?

If your clinic has a policy manual, it should provide you with the answers to questions such as these. Spend some time reviewing the manual, then keep it handy for quick reference.

If you don't have a hospital policy manual, you can make your own. All you need is a notebook labeled "Hospital Policies." Whenever a question of policy arises, make a new heading in your notebook and write down your clinic's policy. If you use a loose-leaf notebook, you can easily arrange your entries in alphabetical order or group them according to subject matter.

Entries might include:

Appointments: Schedule between 9 a.m. and 11:30 a.m. Monday through Friday; 8 a.m. to 1 p.m. on Saturdays.

Phone Calls: Doctor will return routine calls from 11:30 a.m. to 12 p.m. and from 5:30 p.m. to 6 p.m.

Releasing Patients: Doctor will release all hospitalized and surgical cases unless patient chart states otherwise. Make appointments for clients to pick up their pets.

☛ TIP

Receptionists who have worked at other practices may find the above "personalized" hospital policy manual particularly helpful in adjusting to a new employer's system and management style.

Understand Common Medical and Surgical Procedures

"How old should my puppy be before we start her shots?"

"Why does my cat have to stay overnight after he's been declawed?"

"Will my spayed dog still come into heat?"

Understanding the commonly performed medical and surgical procedures at your clinic is a must. You can't these handle questions with confidence until you understand the answers.

Many hospitals write out their puppy and kitten vaccination schedules. (See Chapters 11 and 12.) Keep copies of this information near the phone for quick reference.

As time permits, observe the doctor during routine surgery and dentistry. Ask the doctor to tell you what's being done during the procedure.

Although the number of procedures and treatments seems overwhelming at first, you will find that many are repeated routinely. And so are the clients' questions about them! A question that seems difficult today will be routine to you in a few weeks, so hang in there.

Handling Everyday Details

There is an easy way to keep details from slipping through your fingers: *Pay attention to details and write things down!*

For everything you need to keep track of, you should have a spiral notebook, a status sheet, or an erasable board. Don't trust your memory. *If you don't write it down, you will forget it!* There are simply too many details to remember without help.

Billing Inquiries

All billing inquiries must be resolved. But when a client calls in the morning to ask why he or she received a bill for $10, it's easy to forget about the call as the day progresses. So whenever you have a billing inquiry, reach for your Billing Inquiries notebook. A page in it might look something like this:

Billing Inquiries Note

Date: ______________________________

Client name: ______________________________

Phone number: ______________________________

Nature of query/complaint: ______________________________

Date resolved: ______________________________

How resolved: ______________________________

Even if you can answer a question on the spot, it should be logged in your notebook. You can enter the resolution later. The notebook will show how you handled a question in case a forgetful client calls back a week later to ask the same question!

Outside Lab Work

Outside lab work (lab work that's not done in the clinic) can be tracked the same way. Every time a lab specimen is sent out, it should be logged in an Outside Lab Work notebook. In some hospitals this is the responsibility of the lab technician, but if you are in charge of it at your clinic, you might want to create a form like this:

Outside Lab Work

Date: ______________________

Owner name: ______________________

Phone number: ______________________

Pet name: ______________________

Type of specimen: ______________________

Sent to (name of lab): ______________________

Test(s) requested: ______________________

Results: ______________________

Date received: ______________________

Many labs fax results or provide telephone report forms. Results can be listed there instead of in your notebook. But always note the date the results were received with a notation such as, "Recorded on lab report form," or "See faxed results."

Hospitalized Pets

The condition of hospitalized pets can be listed on a daily status sheet. This will help you handle telephone calls from anxious clients. The doctor may want to fill out the sheet during treatments or may want you to fill it out yourself. The sheet might contain such information as:

Daily Telephone Status Sheet

Owner name: ______________________

Pet name: ______________________

Status: ______________________

Comments: (for example: doctor release, must stay one more day, medication or prescription to fill)

____

____

____

____

If you are part of a large practice with many animals to keep track of, your clinic may already have a master board—usually an erasable board or a chalkboard—that lets you know at a glance which patients are in the clinic and why. The board may be divided into columns. For example:

In-Clinic Status Board

Hospitalized cases	Surgery	Bath	Board
Smith, "Fifi" Hit by car	Jones, "Mitzi" Spay		Johnson, "Rex" through 6/10

A board like this is especially valuable for split shifts. The outgoing receptionist should spend a few minutes going over the board with the incoming receptionist. That way he or she will know the status of every pet that came in during the first shift.

Remember, to be of value, the board must be kept current!

☛ TIP

If you work in a large practice with many hospitalized cases, a Polaroid camera can help you stay organized. Take a picture of each pet as it enters the clinic and tack the picture next to the pet's entry on your master board. This will help eliminate any "who's who" confusion.

Your Desk

Once you have settled in at your new job, you will want to arrange your desk so that everything you need is within easy reach. Things you need every day—your notebooks, for example—should be at your fingertips. Store supplies and things you need only once in a while on top shelves and in cabinets.

A useful tool at the front desk is a Rolodex file with frequently called numbers: animal control, the Society for the Prevention of Cruelty to Animals, the lab, all clinic employees, police, fire, and ambulance. If you have a phone with a memory capability, program important numbers into speed dial and be sure to clearly label each entry.

SUMMARY OF IMPORTANT POINTS

- Organize your references so you'll know where to look for answers to questions.

- Observe hospital surgeries and treatments in order to fully understand them.

- Keep track of queries and other details in writing so you won't forget them and can follow up.

Notes

CHAPTER

3

General Administrative Policies

Should I wear a uniform?
Where did the doctor go to school?
What should I do when a salesperson arrives?

These, and lots of other questions, are answered by your hospital's general administrative policies. Usually these are part of the clinic policy manual, but if your clinic doesn't have a manual (or if it's in need of updating), use this chapter to organize your hospital's policies. Knowing how to handle situations *before* they arise will help you remain calm, collected, and knowledgeable in many different situations.

☛ TIP

Putting your policy manual information on a computer will allow you to easily make changes and print updates.

Know Your Doctors

If you have only one doctor in your practice, this part is easy. If you have more than one, you might want to make a list.

You should know where each doctor went to veterinary school. In addition, you must know each doctor's specialty. Does one of your doctors handle only large animals (horses and cows)? Does one do complex dentistry—root canals, for example? Does one doctor handle all bone surgeries? Are any of the doctors board certified? How many years has each doctor been with the practice?

If all of these questions aren't answered in your clinic's policy manual, reserve a page in one of your notebooks and mark it with a tab. Create a form to fill out for each doctor on staff. You might want it to read like this:

Doctor Information

Name of doctor: ____________________

Veterinary school: ____________________

Year joined practice: ____________________

Specialty (if any): ____________________

Continuing education/special training seminars attended: ____________________

____

Board certified? ____________________

☛ TIP

This is good information to include on your clinic's Web site or in a clinic brochure or folder that is handed out to all new clients. If your clinic doesn't have either one, talk to the doctors about creating one or both. (See Chapter 9.)

Giving Out Home Phone Numbers

Because you are in charge of handling emergencies (see Chapter 7), you have access to the doctors' home phone numbers and beeper numbers. But do the doctors want these numbers kept private, or is it all right to give them to clients who ask for them?

Many doctors, after putting in a long day at the hospital, prefer to let the local emergency clinic (usually open all night) handle after-hours emergencies and monitor critically ill patients overnight.

First, ask the doctors whether they want you to give out their numbers. If not, learn the after-hours care alternatives the doctor recommends that are available in your area. Then be ready to handle those situations that always seem to happen right at closing time.

◆ SAMPLE SITUATION

Mrs. Brown calls 15 minutes before closing, frantic because her dog has been hit by a car. She is on her way to your clinic.

You tell her, *"Mrs. Brown, if Spike is seriously injured, he may need medical attention throughout the night. Dr. Smith recommends that you take him to the emergency clinic. Are you familiar with where it is?"*

Mrs. Brown: *"Yes, I know where it is, but I want Dr. Smith to look at Spike. She's his regular doctor."*

You say: *"You can bring Spike*

to us at 8 o'clock tomorrow morning if he still needs attention. But the best thing for him tonight is to be at the fully staffed emergency clinic. I'll call them and tell them to expect you."

If your area does not have an emergency clinic, the doctors probably take turns being on call. If this is the case, always know which doctor is on call (it may even be a doctor from another practice, especially in the case of large-animal emergencies). This way, you can provide the client with the correct name and phone number.

It is important to be sure the client understands that after-hours care arrangements provide the best possible care for a sick or injured pet. That's why you send them there—*not* because the doctor doesn't care about the client or isn't interested in emergencies that happen after the clinic closes.

If an animal has been hospitalized at your clinic during the day and will be going home for the night, an anxious owner may worry about caring for the pet at home and ask you for the doctor's phone number in case "something happens." Your response would be the same as above: "We don't expect you to have any problems overnight, but if you're unsure about Spike's condition, please call the emergency clinic at this number. They are fully staffed and open all night. Dr. Smith or I will call them about Spike's treatment. That way, if you do need to call them, they'll be familiar with his case."

If the client still seems worried, ask the doctor to place a call during the evening or ask permission to call the client yourself to check on the pet.

Transferring Records

When clients move their pets from your practice to another, they will usually request copies of their pets' records. Because this is usually a permanent transfer, you will need to print out (or photocopy) each pet's entire medical record. If you include fees on your medical records, ask the doctor if the fees should be removed before you transfer the records. Then find out if it is all right to give the records directly to the client or if they should be mailed to the new clinic. Also ask the doctor if he or she needs to make any special notes about the pet's condition.

☛ TIP

It is helpful to go through the records and highlight vaccination dates and important surgeries, such as a spay or neuter.

Most clients request records because they are moving to another location, but occasionally you may have a client who is unhappy with your services (see Chapter 8). In such a case, you would copy the records as described above, but be sure to let the doctor know about the problem. Often, the doctor will want to call or write to the client to see if there is a way to resolve the problem.

Referrals

A referral involves sending ("referring") an animal to a doctor for a one-time procedure, such as a complex surgery or medical treatment. If, for example, a doctor at your clinic specializes in surgically pinning broken bones, animals may be referred to your clinic for this procedure.

If your practice takes referrals, you should know the clinic's policies on accepting incoming patients. For example:

- Does the pet need certain vaccinations? If so, which ones?
- Is the client required to provide the pet's complete medical records?
- Should the client bring X-rays and lab work results or will they be done at your clinic?
- What is the cost of the procedure? What are your payment policies in emergency cases? (See Chapter 5.)
- How long does the pet have to be hospitalized for the procedure?
- Will the pet stay at your practice for follow-up treatment or return to its own veterinarian?

That's a lot to keep track of! Tab a page in your notebook and take the time to jot down the answers to all of the above questions. Also ask your doctor about any other requirements for referrals.

Occasionally this procedure will be reversed, and your doctor will refer a client to another doctor for a procedure or surgery. You may be asked to copy the medical records for the client.

If the client is unhappy or doesn't understand why "her usual doctor" can't do the procedure, explain that the other doctor specializes in this procedure. Perhaps special equipment is needed. Reassure the client that the pet will be back in the care of your clinic very soon. It's important that the client understands that your clinic is making the referral recommendation because you want the pet to have the best possible care!

Salespeople and Solicitors

You already know that an important part of your job is to keep the waiting room organized and the traffic flowing smoothly. So how do you handle unexpected interruptions by salespeople who insist on talking to the doctor or giving you their pitch?

The doctors will usually want to talk to representatives of drug companies so that they can place their orders. In fact, many sales reps make appointments in advance for this purpose. If a salesperson drops in unexpectedly, get his or her business card and see if the doctor has time for the visit. If the doctor is busy, let the salesperson know how long the wait will be, offering the option of waiting or coming back at an appointed time.

To handle other solicitors, find out your doctors' preferences. One doctor may want you to find out what they're selling; another might want you to turn away all solicitors. If solicitors aren't accepted, post a sign that clearly explains your clinic's policy. This should help you discourage salespeople from taking up valuable time and space in the reception area.

Personal Safety

Guidelines for personal safety should be covered your first week on the job. The Occupational Safety and Health Administration (OSHA) sets rules governing safety standards and practices in the workplace, and all new employees must be advised of these rules. You should receive your OSHA training early in your employment, and you should always know where your OSHA manual is. This manual lists hazardous chemicals that could be found in the workplace, how to handle them, and the correct procedures to follow if an employee is overexposed to or harmed by one of these chemicals.

Fire drills should be practiced regularly. Every employee should know the procedure to follow in case of fire, as well as the location and proper use of the fire extinguishers.

Other safety issues that should be addressed early in your employment include:

- Unruly, aggressive, or intoxicated clients in the waiting room. Do you escort them to an exam room? Alert the doctor or another staff member? Call 911?
- Someone trying to rob the clinic. Do you hand over the money? Is there a safety alarm?

When an unexpected situation arises, try to handle it using the guidelines the doctors have established. If the situation is new, use your best judgement and ask the doctors later how they would like you to handle similar situations in the future.

☛ TIP

Any time a question of policy arises, jot it down to talk over with the doctors. Then add it to your policy manual.

Attire and Speech

You will learn if you will wear a uniform as soon as you are hired. If so, does the clinic provide the uniform, or do you need to buy one? If you will not be wearing a uniform, ask about the dress code. Are blue jeans acceptable, or should you wear slacks or a skirt? What about T-shirts and shorts? Are open-toe shoes and shoes with raised heels OK? Should you wear a lab coat over your clothes?

Different positions at the clinic may require different dress codes. Certainly, as the receptionist, you should appear neat and well-groomed at all times.

In addition, speak distinctly and slowly enough that clients have no trouble understanding you. As we mentioned in Chapter 1, you are the clinic's communication link with the outside world. Be sure clients have no trouble understanding you!

SUMMARY OF IMPORTANT POINTS

• Learn your hospital's policies as soon as possible. This will avoid misunderstandings and help you do your job better.

• Make note of new situations and talk them over with the doctor later. When you make a new policy, add it to the manual.

Notes

CHAPTER

4

Answering Clients' Questions

"My dog has been lying around and not eating much of anything for a couple of days. What do you think is wrong?"

For the umpteenth time today, you are being asked to diagnose an illness over the phone. What is the proper way to handle these questions?

You're Not the Doctor, but You Get the Same Questions

Most questions you'll be asked concern everyday matters, such as vaccinations and heartworm tests, and you will be able to answer these types of client queries without consulting the doctor. An overview of medical information and hospital procedures is provided in Chapters 10 through 16 of this manual to help build your knowledge base about routine treatments and procedures. And Chapters 17 and 18 list commonly asked questions along with appropriate responses to each query.

To answer routine questions, you must have a working knowledge of your clinic's vaccination policies and spay and neuter policies (see Chapter 2).

There are three basic categories of routine questions: when, why, and how.

"When" Questions

"When do I start my puppy's shots?"
"When should I neuter my cat?"
"When should my dog start heartworm prevention?"

Clinic policy will answer most "when" questions. If you were thorough in getting organized, you'll know where to find answers to most "when" questions. (See Chapters 11 through 18.)

☛ TIP

When you don't know the answer to a question, tell the caller that you want to be sure to answer the question properly and that you'll call back soon with the answer. Confirm the number to call and then write yourself a note—be sure to return the call!

"Why" Questions

"Why does my pet need a rabies shot every year?"

"Why is it a good idea to spay my cat?"

"I don't see any worms. Why do you need to check under a microscope?"

People want to understand what is best for their pets and why they must spend their hard-earned money. In answering "why" questions, you must communicate the value of a service in a way the client can understand. Never become defensive or say that a certain procedure must be done because it is "hospital policy." If you say, "It must be done," many people will dig in their heels and say, "No, it must not." It's better to relate the value of a service to their own health and medical expenses.

◆ SAMPLE SITUATION

"Why does my dog need to get a distemper shot every year?"

You reply: *"Unfortunately, distemper is still a real problem in our area. We see several cases of distemper each year, and we don't want to risk a possible fatal outcome if your pet catches it. For this reason, the doctor wants to maintain a high level of immunity in your pet. He achieves this by vaccinating your pet each year."*

"Why" questions offer an excellent opportunity for role-playing. Practice your answers with other staff members, and try to get the doctor involved as much as possible so everyone learns together.

"How" Questions

"How do I control fleas?"
"How do I keep my cat from clawing the furniture?"
"How do I housebreak my puppy?"

Your experience gained on the job and with your own pets will help you answer "how" questions. Did you have luck housebreaking your last puppy using a certain method? If so, pass the information along. People always want to hear about methods that have worked for others.

Of course, you won't have experience with every problem that comes up. If your clinic has brochures dealing with various pet problems, give clients those that relate to the pets' problems. If the client is on the phone, offer to mail the brochure.

☛ TIP

Before mailing a brochure to a client, be sure to personalize it. Attach a note saying, for example, "Mr. Brown, I think you'll find the information on Page 3 helpful.

If you continue to have problems with Fluffy, please don't hesitate to call us."

"How" questions that cannot be handled by experience or brochures can often be answered by clinic policy. Most clinics, for example, provide set guidelines to help clients control intestinal parasite outbreaks. Refer to your clinic's guidelines for answers to many of these types of questions.

Medical Questions That Aren't Routine

Let's get back to the question that started this chapter: "What do you think is wrong with my pet?" "What" questions—or any questions that ask for a diagnosis—must be handled properly. When you are in such a situation, use the following guidelines (in this order) to handle the client's question:

1. Ask the client to make an appointment to bring in the pet. You might say, "Mr. Long, from what you are telling me over the phone, I think the doctor should see Spotty. May I make an appointment for you?" (See Chapter 6 on scheduling appointments.) Most clients will choose to schedule an appointment. But sometimes clients won't want to bring their pets in because they may not think the condition is serious enough or may not have the money or time. If a client won't make an appointment:

2. Get the doctor's recommendations after explaining the situation and call the client back with the information. Whenever you do this, pull the client's record and record the date, the client's description of the pet's ailment, what the doctor recommended, and the fact that you conveyed the information to the client.

3. Ask the doctor to return the client's call. Use

your best judgment here. If the problem sounds complicated or the client acts upset, it is often best to let the doctor handle it. Pull the patient's file, attach the client's message with the signs the client described, and give it to the doctor to return the call.

Any time a client calls about a sick pet, the situation should be resolved as quickly as possible. Emergencies are handled immediately, of course. (See Chapter 7.)

If the doctor cannot return a call right away, call the client back yourself and explain that the doctor is in surgery or treating patients and hasn't forgotten the client's question. If you can give the client a definite time the doctor will call back, do so. Remember, if a client is worried enough to call, then a problem exists. The situation should be handled quickly to calm the anxious client and to provide proper treatment for the pet.

➤ POINT TO PONDER

Even if clinical symptoms have been described to you many times, don't diagnose over the phone. Don't recommend medicine and remedies over the phone. There could be unfortunate consequences if you are wrong. You can safely recommend basic first aid—such as direct pressure to stop bleeding—but when in doubt, let the doctor handle it!

Answering Questions About Hospitalized Pets

Clients often will call to check on the condition of hospitalized pets. As we noted in Chapter 2, keep a status report on hospitalized cases or updated files to refer to when answering these questions.

If you're not sure about the condition of a pet, don't guess! It would be unfortunate to report improvement of a pet's condition when in fact it had taken a turn for the worse. Always be sure of your facts. If you are in doubt, call the client back with the information or ask the doctor to do so.

➤ POINT TO PONDER

Medical records are confidential. Details of a patient's treatment (or a client's credit history) should not be given to anyone but the client under any circumstances.

SUMMARY OF IMPORTANT POINTS

- Always be courteous, and use common sense when answering clients' questions. Never volunteer medical advice unless you have checked with the doctor first.

- Always answer the client's question even if you must research the answer and call the client back.

- The more questions you can answer, the less often you will have to interrupt the doctor for answers to routine questions. Interrupt only with emergencies.

Notes

CHAPTER

5

Fee and Payment Policies

How Much Will It Cost?

Many of the questions you will answer each day will concern the cost of your clinic's services. Remember, all price shoppers are potential clients!

➤ POINT TO PONDER

You will be the first person clients meet when they go to your clinic. What you tell them and how you communicate are often the deciding factors in whether they choose your clinic.

Who Are Price Shoppers?

What do we know about someone who calls your clinic and asks the price of a service? Even if the person is a total stranger, we already know two very important things:

1. The caller has a pet.
2. The caller is going to spend money at a veterinary clinic.

It's your job to sell callers on your clinic's ability to help their pets. You must be able to help them understand the value of the services provided at your clinic.

Communicating Value

Giving out price information is much more involved than knowing the cost of a rabies vaccination or the spaying operation—you need to help the client understand the *value* of the service. How do you communicate value?

If you walked into a store and found a shirt you

liked, you would ask the sales clerk how much it was. If the clerk looked at you and said, "$95," you might think, "Wow, that's really expensive," and walk out of the store.

But if the sales clerk said that the shirt was 100 percent pure silk, washable, handmade, and could be worn year round, and *then* quoted the same price, you might think, "That's a good value."

One of your most important jobs as veterinary receptionist is to communicate value. You must make clients understand why the services are priced the way they are and why the clients will be getting good value. Anyone can quote a price over the telephone. It's your job to make clients feel they are getting top value even though they may be spending more money at your clinic than they would at another veterinary hospital.

◆ SAMPLE SITUATION

A client calls and asks how much it will cost to have his dog spayed.

You say, *"Mr. Smith, at our clinic the price includes the hospitalization of your pet, the presurgical exam, the anesthesia, the actual surgery with vital signs monitored at all times, close observation during recovery, and continued checks until your pet goes home. For your size dog, the price would be $95."*

"Well," thinks Mr. Smith, *"they do all that for my pet for $95. That's a good value."*

In the example above, not only has value been communicated, but the client will see that the pet will receive the staff's full attention during its stay in the hospital.

It is an excellent idea to "role play" what you will say when communicating value—not to the point where you have a stiff, memorized speech, but just so you're comfortable with what you are saying. The more comfortable you are, the more confident you'll sound and the better you will get your point across. Ask the other clinic employees to role play with you—they may have additional suggestions.

Once you are comfortable with the idea of communicating value, you should get down to the "nuts and bolts" of your clinic's prices and learn the fee structure.

Learning Your Clinic's Fee Structure

Most clinics keep a list of services and fees at the front desk. If you are a new staff member at your practice, be sure that the prices are up to date. Quoting an old price will only cause misunderstanding when it is time for the client to pay the bill.

Don't panic! You don't need to memorize every price on the list. But you should learn the prices for the most commonly performed services. For example, you will often be asked about the prices for routine vaccinations, spaying, and neutering. You should also know the price of an office visit.

☛ TIP

When new clients call your office to compare prices, ask them to give you their names and addresses so that you can mail them information about your clinic or about the services they asked about. This helps acquaint them with your clinic and could help make them regular clients.

You might find it helpful to make a chart of puppy, kitten, and adult vaccinations (if your clinic doesn't already have one) and keep it handy until you're familiar with each of these visits. On it you would list what services the pet receives, what each service costs, and the total for the entire visit.

For example:

Puppy, 6 to 9 Weeks Old

First distemper/parvo vaccine	$9
First corona vaccine	$6
Fecal check	$10
Physical exam	$25
Total cost:	$50
(plus $6 for deworming if needed)	

What to Do When You Don't Know the Price

People often want to know prices only the doctor can quote. For example, a client may call and say his or her dog has been hit by a car and ask you the cost of fixing the dog's broken leg.

Because this type of injury can involve X-rays, medication, hospitalization, a splint, or bone surgery, you will not be able to quote a price over the phone. The best way to handle this is to say, "From what you are telling me, Mrs. Smith, I think the doctor should see your dog. Our office visit is $25, and when the doctor examines your pet, he will be able to give you an accurate estimate of the cost. May I make an appointment for you?"

Payment Policies

Animal hospitals are not lending institutions. Therefore, the payment policy of most is very simple:

Fees are due when services are rendered.

Ideally, all fees should be collected at the time of the service. Many clinics offer a variety of payment methods to accommodate their clients, including cash, personal checks, and credit cards.

You might want to highlight the methods your clinic accepts on a sign at the front desk.

Payment by Cash

This is the easiest type of payment to handle because no verification is necessary. It simply requires that you count the cash carefully, both in accepting payment and in making change.

Always give the client a receipt. With a cash sale, the receipt will be the client's only proof of purchase.

Payment by Check

Most clinics accept only personal checks—that means only those checks written on the client's personal account, made payable to your clinic.

Second-party checks (those written to the client by another person), payroll checks, and other nonpersonal checks are usually not acceptable forms of payment.

When accepting a personal check from a client, verify the client's name, address, and phone number as it appears on the check. Note any differences between the information on the check and the information in the client's file. If there is a difference, determine which is correct. If the client has given you a post office box number only, get a street address as well. Write the client's driver's license number and work phone number on the check.

☛ TIP

Keep a driver's license number and work phone number in every client's file so you won't have to write them on the check at each visit.

Some other things to keep in mind about accepting checks include:

1. Never accept a check that is post-dated, not dated, or more than 10 days old.
2. Be sure the check is signed.
3. Make sure the numerical figure agrees with the amount written on the check.

If a check is returned to you because there are insufficient funds in the check writer's account, ask him or her to pick up the bad check and give you cash for it. Because you'll need to know where to find the person who wrote the check, obtain a home address and work number from every client. If you are unable to contact the client, the Division of Motor Vehicles will provide you with the client's last known address if you tell them the client's driver's license number.

If your clinic uses an electronic check-approval service, you will probably be required to call and verify all checks over a certain amount. Make a note of your hospital's guidelines in the box that follows.

If you do not have such a service and you are in doubt about the worth of a check, you can call the bank named on the check to verify it. This should not be done in the client's presence. Simply excuse yourself by saying you have to get check approval, and privately make the phone call. A bank's bookkeeping department won't tell you a client's balance, but it will tell you whether a check for a certain amount will clear.

Use the space below to make notes on your clinic's policy on accepting checks.

Clinic Policy on Accepting Checks

Personal checks accepted: Yes No

Second-party (other non-personal checks) accepted: Yes No

Type of verification required:

Under $50 ________________.

Over $50 __________________.

Approval of ______________ also required for checks over $________.

Call ____________ to verify all checks over $ ______.
(phone number)

Payment by Credit Card

When accepting a credit card payment, verify the name on the card and the card's expiration date. If you have an electronic credit card processing terminal in your office, it will automatically verify the credit card, print a receipt, and deposit the money in the clinic's bank account.

If you use a manual processing system, learn your clinic's policy on verifying charges over a certain amount. Post the phone number to call for verification, unless your verification system automatically dials the number. Use the space below for your clinic's policy on charge card verification:

Clinic Policy on Charge Card Verification

Call to verify all charges over:

$ _____ for Master Card Phone __________

$ _____ for Visa Phone __________

$ _____ for Am. Express Phone __________

$ _____ for ________ (other) Phone __________

☛ TIP

Always get phone verification before handing the card and the completed charge slip back to the client. If authorization for the charge is denied, you will want the client to be in the clinic so you can request that the client use another method of payment.

Once verification is complete, ask the client to sign the charge slip, then give him or her a copy and a clinic receipt.

Exceptions to the Payment Rule

Now that we have described ideal payment policies, let's take a look at not-so-ideal payment situations. There are always people who, for one reason or another, do not pay at the time of service. This should happen *only when the client has made arrangements in advance with the doctor* and the doctor has approved the charge.

Clients who have permission to be billed later should have their records flagged or coded in some way to let you know their charge has been approved (and to save everyone embarrassment at the checkout counter). Otherwise, no one should leave your clinic without paying for services.

NOTE: There is a difference between emergency and elective services when it comes to payment policies. Although payment is always due, unforeseen emergencies can sometimes stretch a family's budget to the breaking point. (See Chapter 7.) There is no reason, however, for a client to postpone paying for such elective procedures as vaccinations, spaying, and neutering. These procedures could be done at any time—for example, when the client has set aside enough money to pay for them at the time the service is rendered.

Although it's easy to say that no client should

leave without paying for services, this is sometimes difficult to enforce. Let's look at a few examples.

"I Don't Have the Money"

A client has just spent half an hour with the doctor. He presents himself at your desk. You say, "That will be $52, Mr. Long." Mr. Long says, "I don't have enough money to pay that. Can you bill me?" What do you do? Here are some examples of how to handle the situation, depending on your clinic's policy.

- First ask if he would like to put it on his credit card.
- If he has no credit card, stay calm, smile, and say, "That's fine, Mr. Long. Go ahead and make out a check with today's date, and I'll put a note for the bookkeeper to deposit it on the day of your choice."
- Or you might say, "That's fine. Go ahead and divide the amount in half, write two checks dated today and tell me what day you would like each check deposited."

When a client has written a check and given it to you, that money is committed in the client's mind, and therefore can't spend it on something else. If the client leaves without giving you a check, you may have trouble collecting it later.

☛ TIP

Clients who do not intend to pay frequently become loud and disruptive. (See Chapter 8 for tips on handling the "unhappy client.")

NOTE: From a legal standpoint, you will have little recourse if you hold a check as described in the above examples and the check bounces. In effect, you admitted that you knew there were insufficient funds in the client's account when you agreed to accept the check, and therefore you should not be surprised when it bounces. *Check with the doctor to see if holding a check is an acceptable payment policy at your clinic before using it.*

Another option is a third-party check that is kept in escrow until the bill is paid in full, whether all at once or in installments. In effect, the held check is a guarantee and an agreement of trust. You trust the client to pay the bill in full by the designated time, and the client trusts you to hold the check until payment is complete. When the bill is paid, the client receives the returned check, along with a signed and dated statement from the clinic noting that the check was returned. As with other alternative payment plans, be sure that all terms of the agreement are put in writing.

☛ TIP

When handling a collection problem, be pleasant but firm and assertive—never bullying, aggressive, or sarcastic. And don't involve the doctor unless absolutely necessary. Take the attitude, "This is our policy and I am responsible for enforcing it."

"I Forgot My Checkbook"

Let's look at the above example but change Mr. Long's answer to "I forgot my checkbook" or "I don't have a checking account." Now, rather than not having enough money, the client has no way to pay the bill at all.

First ask if the charge could be put on a credit card. If that fails, follow these procedures:

• If the client is one whom you know and trust, put the bill in an envelope addressed to your clinic and ask the client to mail it with a check. If your clinic charges a billing fee after a certain number of days, that should be noted on the bill as well. Be sure you explain this policy to the client.

• New clients or those whom you don't know shouldn't leave the clinic until they have agreed *in writing* to make full payment by a certain date. Many clinics have standard payment-plan forms or promissory notes which you can fill out and have the client sign. In filling out one of these forms, take the following precautions:

1. Verify the spelling of the client's first and last name.
2. Double-check the address. Be sure that it is the address where the client receives mail. If it is a rural route or a post office box, also get a street address.
3. Verify the client's phone number with area code. Always get a work number as well as the actual place of employment. If the client has no work number, try to get the number of a relative or neighbor.
4. Ask to see the client's driver's license. Record the number and expiration date. Check the name and address on the license, and be sure it corresponds to your files.
5. Note the total amount due and the manner in which the client will pay it. For example, if the bill is $52, write on the note that the entire sum will be paid by the fifteenth of the month or that the client will pay $10 a week until the balance is paid by a specific date.

6. If interest charges will be applied, figure them into the payment amounts on the note, and be sure the client understands the amounts and the dates on which payment is due.

7. Have the client sign and date the agreement, then have someone who represents the clinic sign it as well.

8. Give the client one copy and keep one copy for your files.

☛ TIP

Figuring and writing payment plans and promissory notes takes a considerable amount of time and thought, especially when the client is standing impatiently at the checkout counter. You can avoid some of the time-consuming complications if you determine how the client plans to pay for the services rendered ***before the doctor sees the pet.***

New clients should note on the registration form how they intend to pay. Be sure each new client checks a payment method or is asked how the visit will be paid for. This lets you avoid many unfortunate situations before they ever reach the payment counter.

NOTE: Alternative payment plans, such as the promissory note described above, should *not* be offered as payment options. Clients who ask to be billed should be told that payment is due when services are rendered. Explain the payment methods your clinic offers, which could include cash, checks, or credit cards.

☛ TIP

Code or tag the files of clients who have a history of presenting collection problems and being slow in paying their bills. This will help you avoid problems by alerting you the moment you pull the file. It also will help the doctor know if the client might present a problem—especially if he or she is meeting the client alone to treat an emergency.

It is important to keep in mind that money is a touchy subject with many people. Having to part with it can bring out the worst in them. Always remain pleasant when payment problems arise, and don't feel you have to defend your clinic's prices or policies or sympathize that a bill is too high. As a rule, the cost of veterinary services is one of the last true bargains available in our society.

Ideally, the client was given an estimate before treatment began and has been kept up to date with the cost of treatment as it progressed. As we said earlier, clients will not, in general, resent the cost of services if they *perceive that the value of the services is equal to the cost that has been charged.*

SUMMARY OF IMPORTANT POINTS

- Keep a price list handy, and quote prices carefully and accurately. If you don't know the price of something, find out and call the client back.
- Always collect fees at the time of the client's visit or when the pet is discharged from the hospital.
- If a client is unable to pay, a written payment agreement should be made before the client leaves the clinic.

Notes

CHAPTER 6

Scheduling Appointments

A carefully maintained appointment system keeps the clinic running smoothly. It allows time for the doctor to complete treatments and perform surgery, and it prevents a pile-up in the waiting room and unpleasantly long waits for the clients.

Turning Question Calls Into Appointments

Many of the calls you receive each day will be from people who want you to diagnose their pets' ailments over the phone. These calls are generally from people who are "too busy" to make a trip to the veterinarian or whose monetary situation makes a visit impossible at the time.

The first group can often be converted into appointments by saying pleasantly—remember your golden rule—"Mrs. Smith, from what you are describing to me over the phone, it sounds like something the doctor should see. Would later today be convenient for you?"

Remember, nearly every phone call that comes into the clinic regarding a change in a pet's normal habits or functions may be the beginning of something serious. It is always better to make an appointment so that the doctor can examine the pet and make a diagnosis.

A client who feels uneasy enough about abnormal behavior to call needs to come in. It is much better to treat a vomiting puppy while it is still strong than to have it go into convulsions and then try to treat it.

Also, most doctors would prefer to see their clients during regular office hours rather than in the middle of the night!

(See Chapter 5 for information on converting price-shopping calls into appointments.)

Making an Accurate Appointment

Information You Need

Every time you make an appointment, you should be sure to obtain the following information about the client and the pet:

1. the client's name
2. the pet's name and species
3. whether the client is new or has visited the clinic before
4. the client's phone number—this is very important; you may have to call the client back to reschedule the appointment
5. the purpose of the visit
6. which, if any, of the doctors the client would prefer to schedule an appointment with (if the clinic is a multiple-doctor practice)

Appointment Book Entry

Helen Johnston (new)
"Rex," dog, yearly vaccination
555-1212
Dr. Hanson

☛ TIP

If you keep a record of your clinic's appointments on the computer, remember to print several copies of the schedule each day. Then give a copy to the doctors, the technicians, the kennel help, and yourself.

Information the Client Needs

The client who has made the appointment also needs certain information from you. Before you hang up the phone, be sure the client knows:

1. where the clinic is located
2. the time to arrive (new clients may have to arrive a few minutes early to fill out forms)
3. special instructions for the appointment (bring a stool sample, do not feed your pet before the visit, etc.)

☛ TIP

When scheduling appointments over the phone, always repeat the day and time of the appointment, using both the client's and pet's names. Any confusion that can be cleared up over the telephone will save time and trouble in the waiting room.

Some clients may resist making an appointment at first. They often feel they can't be pinned down to a certain time. It is your job to help these clients understand the advantages of scheduling an appointment.

◆ SAMPLE SITUATION

The telephone rings.

You answer the phone promptly and cheerfully: *"Good morning. Main Street Animal Clinic. This is Linda. How may I help you?"*

Caller: *"Hi Linda. This is Mark Johnson. I'd like to bring my dog in today for some shots. Would just about any time be OK to see the doctor?"*

You clarify the purpose of the client's visit: *"Mr. Johnson, is your dog due for its annual vaccinations?"*

Caller: *"Yes, that's right. I got a reminder card from you. So I'll be in some time today. What time do you close?"*

You: *"The doctor has a busy schedule today, and I wouldn't want you to have a long wait when you come. May I set up an appointment for you so we can get you in and out quickly?"*

The client will usually agree because a long wait with an anxious dog is not a happy prospect for anyone. You then agree on a time and get the necessary information from the client.

When to Schedule Appointments

Obviously you can't schedule appointments from morning until night every day of the week, or there wouldn't be time for the doctor to do anything else.

Each doctor has preferences concerning appointment hours, surgery time, farm calls, lunch break, and time devoted to paperwork.

Duty Schedule for Multiple-Doctor Practice

Hours to schedule appointments: ______________________

Days/hours to schedule farm calls: ______________________

No appointments on (day): ______________________

from (time): ______________________

to (time): ______________________

Special notes: ______________________

For example, "No baths or dips on Saturday." "No surgery on Wednesday morning."

To accustom yourself to the hospital schedule, fill in the chart above and keep it posted near the appointment book.

You will also need to know how much time the doctor requires for each appointment. This will vary according to the purpose of the visit. Fill in the following chart (as shown in the first example) with your doctor's preferences.

Time Allotment for Clinic Services				
	Schedule in		Minutes	Special
Purpose of visit	**a.m.**	**p.m.**	**to allow**	**instructions**
Annual vacc (dog – sample)	X	X	20	Bring stool sample
Annual vacc (cat)				
First puppy visit				
First kitten visit				
Follow–up puppy visits				
Follow–up kitten visits				
Exam—sick pet				
Doctor release surgery				
Doctor release hospitalized pet				
Stitch removal				
Clip nails				
X-ray				
Heartworm check only				
Fecal check only				
FeLV test only				
Bath and dip				

☛ TIP

It is often a good idea to leave 10 minutes open during each hour for the doctor to see emergencies, sick pets of regular clients who call at the last minute, or simply to catch up when things are busy.

Clients often want to know how much the visit will cost at the time they make the appointment. See Chapter 5 on familiarizing yourself with your clinic's fee structure and on how to communicate value when quoting prices.

☛ TIP

Knowing how much time to allow for each appointment will help only if you remember to ask each client the purpose of the visit! Be sure you know why the client is scheduling an appointment.

Scheduling Vaccination Appointments

Filling out the appointment-times chart gives you a good idea how long a vaccination appointment will take. But that is only part of what you need to know.

When a client calls for a vaccination appointment, ask whether the pet is having any problems that need the doctor's attention. If a pet has an allergy, for example, a routine 20-minute appointment could easily stretch into 40 minutes. So try to determine *everything* that will need to be done while the pet is at the clinic.

Ask the client to bring a stool sample. Most yearly vaccinations include a fecal check for intestinal parasites. A good way to phrase this request is, "Your pet's visit would be more thorough if you could bring a stool sample."

If time permits, pull the client's chart while you're on the phone together and see if any other pets are due for vaccination. Many clients would rather get all their pets vaccinated in one trip.

Scheduling Appointments for Sick Pets

Appointments for sick pets should be made as soon as your schedule permits—the sooner the better! In order to schedule the right amount of time, try to determine the nature of the pet's illness. If a cat swallowed something, the doctor may need to have X-rays taken. If a dog is vomiting, it may need to be seen immediately.

If a pet has diarrhea or intestinal upset, ask the owner to bring a stool sample. The doctor may want to rule out parasites in making a diagnosis.

If the pet ate something (poison or medicine, for example) ask the owner to bring it so the doctor can determine exactly what course of treatment to pursue.

NOTE: Cases of acute poisoning are considered emergencies. See Chapter 7 for details.

Be sure to instruct the client not to give the pet any medicine at home unless the doctor gives other instructions. Home medication can often mask the pet's clinical signs.

Scheduling Surgery and Dentistry

How Much to Schedule

Large hospitals with many doctors may schedule surgery every day and still maintain a full appointment schedule. Smaller practices with one doctor may set aside a few hours each day for surgery. Other clients will not be scheduled during the time the doctor is performing surgery.

Whichever type of practice you work for, it is important to know how much surgery to schedule and when to schedule it.

Because some surgeries may take 10 minutes and others may take more than an hour, it's not enough to say, "I can schedule three surgical procedures every day." You must know how much time the doctor plans to spend in surgery and how many surgeries it will take to fill up that time.

Let the doctor tell you how to schedule surgeries according to his or her preferences—spays one day, neuters another day, and ear crops on a different day, for example.

Surgeries may also be scheduled by time. If two hours a day are scheduled for surgery, you will need to know how long each procedure takes and schedule accordingly. For example, if a large-dog spay takes 50 minutes, a cat spay 30 minutes, and an ear trim 40 minutes, those three surgeries would fill the two hours. Complete the first three columns of the chart on page 75 according to your doctor's preference. This will help you schedule surgery accurately and efficiently.

What You Need to Know About the Pet

To fill in the fourth column of the chart, ask your doctor about vaccination, fecal, and heartworm requirements for surgical cases. Many doctors require that pets be current on all vaccinations and be tested negative for intestinal parasites before routine, elective surgery can be performed. In addition, dogs must usually be on heartworm-prevention medication or test negative for heartworms.

When you make a surgical appointment, pull the file to check that all vaccinations are current. Ask new clients if everything is current, and, if possible, verify it with their previous veterinarians.

Ask about the size of the pet. Large dogs often take more time than small dogs. Is the pet in heat or pregnant? Does it have nursing puppies or kittens? All of these affect the surgery, and all are discussed in more detail in Chapter 15.

What the Client Needs to Know

The fifth column of our surgery chart is for information you need to convey to the client.

For example, most surgical patients must come in on an empty stomach because anesthesia can cause stomach upset. Therefore, you may have to tell a client not to feed the pet the night before or the morning of the surgery.

It is also a good idea to have the client give the pet a flea bath the day before surgery. This kills external parasites and cleans the pet. In areas where fleas and ticks are a problem, this is a must and often will be done at the clinic (for a fee) the morning of the surgery.

Different surgical procedures have different requirements. Use your surgical chart to remind you of the proper things to tell each client. When the pet comes in for surgery, be sure to get a phone number where the client can be reached during the day. Reassure the client by explaining, "This is in case the doctor has any questions or finds anything else that needs immediate attention."

Making the Appointment

When you make an appointment for surgery or dentistry, be sure to get all the information that you would get when making a regular appointment.

In addition, be sure the client knows when to bring the pet in, when to call to check on the pet, and when to pick up the pet.

A typical surgical appointment note might look something like this:

Surgical Appointment

Ann Smith, "Boomer," female dog, 30 lbs., Spay

All vaccinations current, advised to give flea bath

555-9191

☛ TIP

Schedule a release appointment for each pet having surgery. This gives the doctor a few unrushed moments to talk with the client about any special home care, instructions, and any follow-up visits.

Many clinics have printed instructions for post-surgical home care. Whenever you give a client such a handout, be sure to explain what it is and highlight the most important sections. People are more apt to take the time to read something when they know where the important information is and how it pertains to them.

◆ SAMPLE SITUATION

A client calls your office wanting to have her 7-month-old cat spayed.

You say: *"Certainly, Mrs. Smith, we can do that for you this week. Has your cat been to our clinic before?"*

Mrs. Smith: *"Oh, yes, I brought Fluffy to you when she was just a kitten."*

You: *"Good. Then she must be current on her vaccinations—feline distemper, leukemia and rabies. Is that correct?"*

Mrs. Smith: *"Yes, she's had everything she's supposed to have."*

(Pull the client's file to double-check the vaccination status.)

You: *"Would Wednesday morning be a convenient time to bring her in?"*

Mrs. Smith: *"That would be fine."*

You: *"Mrs. Smith, I'd like you to have Fluffy here at 9 o'clock Wednesday morning. Please don't feed her or give her water after 10 o'clock Tuesday night or on Wednesday morning. It's important that her stomach be empty when she goes under anesthesia. Do you have any questions about that?"*

Mrs. Smith: *"No, I understand."*

You: *"Mrs, Smith, are you using a monthly flea and tick prevention on Fluffy?"*

Mrs. Smith: *"No, I'm not."*

You: *"At this time of year all pets are plagued by fleas. We recommend that you give Fluffy a flea bath on Tuesday to have her as clean as possible for her surgery. Will you be able to do this, or would it be more convenient for us to do it Wednesday morning?"*

Mrs. Smith: *"Will it cost extra if you do it?"*

You: *"Our charge for a pre-surgical bath is $6."*

Mrs. Smith: *"I'll do my best to get her bathed on Tuesday."*

You: *"You can call on Wednesday afternoon about 3 o'clock to check on her if you would like, and plan to pick her up at 5:15."*

Mrs. Smith: *"That will be fine. How much is this going to cost?"*

You: *"A routine spay is $65. This includes the presurgical examination, the anesthesia, the* *surgery itself, Fluffy's hospitalization and postsurgical care, and the removal of the stitches next week. If the doctor advises me of any additional charges, I'll call to let you know. You may pay when you pick Fluffy up."*

Scheduling Surgical Procedures

Type of surgery	Minutes to allow	When to schedule	Presurgical vaccination required	Instructions to owner
(Example) Spay cat	40	Any day	All	Withhold food and water after 10 p.m. the night before surgery

Scheduling Large-Animal or Farm Calls

If your practice includes large animals—horses, cows, pigs—you will need to know how to schedule farm calls. Livestock can't always be easily transported to the clinic, especially if an injury or serious illness is involved (see Chapter 7 on the best ways to handle emergencies).

First, find out whether all the doctors handle large animals or if they are one doctor's specialty. Then determine if routine farm calls are made every day or only on certain days. Ask the doctor how much time (including travel time) to allow for various procedures. If you are in doubt about how to schedule a particular procedure, ask!

☛ TIP

Some doctors prefer to make their own farm call appointments. Learn your doctor's preference for large-animal appointments.

When you make the actual appointment, obtain the same information you would for a small animal. If your clinic has large-animal facilities, try to have the client bring the animal to the clinic. It is usually easier to treat an animal at the hospital than in the barn or pasture.

If the doctor must go to the client's house, ask if the doctor has been there before. If in doubt, get directions from the client. And always get a phone number.

☛ TIP

*Always ask the client to catch and pen the animal **before** the doctor makes the call. Precious time can be wasted trying to catch a cow or horse in a large pasture.*

SUMMARY OF IMPORTANT POINTS

- Be sure you understand how long a procedure takes before scheduling an appointment for it. When in doubt, ask!
- Know your doctors' specialties. That way you can schedule certain procedures with the correct doctor.
- Keep a detailed appointment book. It will not only help you prepare for pulling files and filling out consent forms, it will also allow you to reschedule appointments when necessary.

Notes

CHAPTER

7

Handling Emergencies

Emergencies can be a stressful part of working in an animal clinic, with panicked owners, injured pets, and people running in every direction at once. But you don't have to be anxious about emergencies if you prepare for them.

☛ TIP

Handing a "mock" emergency is an excellent topic for a staff meeting. Use your clinic pet, or a rolled up towel, and go through the steps of handling an emergency until everyone is comfortable with the process.

If you practice ahead of time you'll know exactly what steps to take, whether a doctor is there or not. The more prepared you are, the calmer you will be during an actual emergency and the easier it will be for you to take control and handle the situation calmly and professionally. The most important rules for any emergency are:

Stay calm.
Don't panic.
Take control.

A distraught owner is in no position to take control, so you have to. He or she will be looking to you to know what to do. By remaining calm and taking predetermined steps to handle the emergency you will automatically calm the owner.

☛ TIP

Remaining calm and self-assured does not *mean having an indifferent attitude toward a client with an emergency. Remember, you care about your clients' pets as much as they do. Reassure distressed clients by saying, "The doctor will see your pet immediately. One of us will be back to talk with you as soon as your pet has been examined."*

In-Clinic Emergencies

When the Doctor is Present

Your waiting room is full when Mr. Ford rushes in carrying the limp form of his dog. "Tuffy's been hit by a car!" he shouts.

First, don't panic. If you do, you will only increase his fear. Stay in control and immediately take appropriate action—put your emergency plan into effect. A typical emergency drill might be as follows:

1. Get the victim and owner out of the waiting room and into a treatment area.

2. Advise the doctor immediately of the arrival of an emergency, especially if the pet is unconscious or obviously traumatized. In this one instance it is permissible to interrupt a doctor who is with a client, but be sure to do so in a professional manner. For example, "Excuse me, Doctor, but an emergency accident victim has just been brought in. I've taken it to the exam table in the treatment room."

3. The doctor examines the pet and decides whether it needs immediate attention or is stable enough to wait for a few minutes.

4. Separate a panicked owner from the pet. You might try to comfort and reassure the owner in the lounge or an empty exam room, offering a drink of water or cup of coffee. This is a good time to get the client's name and pull the pet's file (or create a new one, if needed).

5. By the time you have finished your paperwork with the client, the doctor will probably be ready to give a brief status report on the pet.

However your doctor chooses to handle emergencies, it is important to have a plan and stick to it. If your doctor has a preferred emergency plan, use the space below to write it down.

Clinic Emergency Plan

☛ TIP

If you're not sure whether it's an emergency, don't guess! Treat it as if it is. It's better to be ready with treatment than to wait until it's too late. Let the doctor examine the pet and make the decision on how urgent the need for treatment is.

The chart at the end of the chapter lists some common emergencies. Use it to familiarize yourself with emergency situations, but don't look up each emergency as it presents itself. And don't dismiss anyone because a particular emergency situation is not listed in the chart—anything can happen to a pet at any time! When in doubt, put your emergency plan into effect.

☛ TIP

Many emergencies have to do with pets getting into poison. Post the number of your local Poison Control Center in a prominent place or program it into your memory dial so you can call quickly when you need to know the antidote to a certain poison.

When the Doctor Is Unavailable

The situation described above can be even more frightening if it happens when the doctor is out of the office. Don't wait until you're alone and have to figure out what to do. Know your clinic's procedures ahead of time.

Some doctors allow their most qualified staff members to administer first aid (stop the bleeding or clear an airway, for example) while a doctor is called or paged.

If the doctor will be unavailable for a long time, you may be required to refer the emergency elsewhere. If that is the case, know whom you are supposed to call and have the number by the phone. Also, be sure you are able to give directions to the designated clinic.

☛ TIP

Any time you must refer an emergency to another clinic, it's important to call ahead to be sure that the doctor is in and will be ready to treat the emergency. You wouldn't want to send your client to another clinic where the doctor is out or is unable to see the patient.

NOTE: Never treat or administer drugs to an animal yourself unless the doctor has given you explicit instructions to do so. Use the space on the next page to outline your emergency procedure when the doctor is out of the office.

Emergency Procedures

Call doctor at: ______________________________ (home)

______________________________ (pager)

If doctor is reached and is on the way, treat the emergency victim as follows:

If doctor cannot be reached, refer emergency to:

Clinic: ____________________________

Address: __________________________

Phone number: ___________________

or to:

Clinic: ____________________________

Address: __________________________

Phone number: ___________________

The After-Hours Emergency

Your clinic closes at 6 p.m. At 5:55 p.m., a client calls and says his dog has been bitten by a snake and it will take him half an hour to get there. What do you do?

Many clinics, especially those with more than one doctor on staff, handle after-hours emergencies themselves. If this is the case in your clinic, you should have a schedule that lists which doctor is on call on any given day. That way, you'll be able to tell the client, "You can bring your pet in immediately. Dr. Brown will be here."

If your clinic charges an emergency fee, you should tell the client about the fee while on the phone.

Other clinics may refer after-hours emergencies to an emergency clinic that is open nights and weekends. Clients sometimes resist being sent elsewhere—they want to see their own doctor and cannot understand why they can't after the clinic has closed.

The best way to avoid the possibility of alienating an anxious client is to say, "Mr. Jones, I know how concerned you are about Sparky, and we're concerned, too. We would feel better if he were at the emergency clinic, where someone could watch him all night. We couldn't do that here. I think it would be best for Sparky to have round-the-clock attention. If the doctor at the emergency clinic feels Sparky will need further treatment, Dr. Brown will see him first thing in the morning."

☛ TIP

Make a note to follow up on emergency cases you have referred elsewhere. A phone call the next day will show how much your clinic cares about the client and about the pet's condition.

Use the space below to outline your clinic's after-hours emergency policies.

After-Hours Emergency Policies

Refer after-hours emergencies to: ______________

Phone: ______________

Refer after-hours emergencies to staff doctor on duty.

Doctors' duty schedule: ______________________

Large-Animal Emergencies

In the middle of a busy morning filled with appointments, the phone rings. Mrs. Jones says, "My mare got into the sweet feed, and now she's colicking. Tell the doctor I need her right away."

Certain large-animal emergencies need immediate attention (see the end of this chapter for a list of some of them), and usually the doctor will have to leave the clinic to tend to them. If your practice has more than one doctor, one can handle the emergency while the others handle appointments. If there is just one doctor, you will need to rearrange the appointments to allow the doctor to tend to the emergency.

If the caller is a regular client, ask which animal is ill and whether the client has a way to transport it to the clinic. If the client can't bring in the animal, assure the client that the doctor will be there as soon as possible. If you don't know the caller, obtain his or her address and phone number as well as directions the house.

☛ TIP

Often the doctor will want to speak to a client whose large animal has an emergency—either to recommend first aid or to determine the severity of the animal's problem. Always give the doctor the option of talking to the client before you hang up.

If the doctor is in surgery or unable to tend to the emergency immediately, he or she may want you to refer the client elsewhere. Handle this just as you would a small-animal emergency referral as described earlier.

Fill in the box on the next page with the appropriate information.

Clinic Procedure for Large-Animal Emergency Referral

If doctor is unavailable, refer large-animal emergencies to:

Name of doctor:	Phone number:
____________________	________________

or to:

Name of doctor:	Phone number:
____________________	________________

Over-the-Phone Emergencies

One of the most common problems with an over-the-phone emergency is persuading the caller to calm down long enough to tell you what is actually wrong with the pet. The first thing to do, then, is to *identify the problem.* Get the caller's name and phone number. Even if you do not think it is a true emergency, arrange to have the client bring the pet to the clinic as soon as possible.

☛ TIP

If the client feels that the situation at hand is an emergency, then it is. The pet should be brought in immediately. The doctor can then evaluate the pet's condition and decide whether the pet needs immediate treatment or could wait for a few minutes.

Always recommend extreme caution in handling an injured pet. Injured animals tend to bite, and the owner may want to muzzle the pet—for example, by tying its mouth shut with a stocking or scarf—before trying to move it. Pets that have been hit by a car should be moved on a sheet of plywood, if possible, to avoid further trauma.

Often there is no time to convey these instructions, and it is important only to get the pet to the clinic. Clients who have no way of getting the pet to the doctor should either ask friends or neighbors for help or call an animal ambulance if one is available in the community.

In extremely urgent situations, the doctor may decide to examine the animal at the client's home. This option is one that the doctor would decide on after talking to the client. It should never be suggested as a routine way of handling emergencies.

Emergency Payment Policies

Extreme situations sometimes require extreme responses. As we said in Chapter 6, every client should pay for services at the time they are rendered. However, a bill of several hundred dollars to fix a broken bone may stretch the budget of some clients and be impossible to pay for others.

Following your emergency drill, you have already separated the owner from the pet. After completing an examination, the doctor may want to talk to the owner about the extent of the injuries and the cost to make the pet well, or he or she might instead work up an estimate and have you discuss the treatment plan and its cost with the client.

The client then faces a difficult decision—to spend the money to make the pet well or to have the doctor perform euthanasia. Whatever the decision, *do not be judgmental.*

If the injuries are severe and the client chooses euthanasia, comfort him or her by saying, "I understand your decision. We will take care of everything and make arrangements for the body if you don't wish to take it home with you."

Be sure that a client choosing euthanasia signs a euthanasia consent form. This preprinted form lists the client's name and address and the pet's name and description. A short statement gives the doctor permission to euthanize the animal. It should be signed and dated by the client and kept as a permanent part of the patient record.

NOTE: No pet should be euthanized without a signed consent form.

A client who chooses medical care should be given an estimate of the total cost. It should be made clear that this is an estimate and that complications could cause the cost to increase. Most doctors want a deposit before they begin treatment, whether the client intends to pay the entire balance at the time of release or not.

If the client will not be able to pay the entire balance at the time of release, he or she should complete a payment plan (described in Chapter 5) before leaving the clinic.

Use the space on the next page to outline your clinic's payment policy in emergency cases:

Clinic Payment Policy for Emergency Cases

Give written estimate:	___ Yes	___ No
Have client leave deposit:	___ Yes	___ No
Payment plan completed and signed:	___ Yes	___ No

Other guidelines: ______________________________

____

☛ TIP

Many emergency victims will be first-time clients. Be sure to get complete information on each client (name, address, phone number, work number) at the time of treatment. This may be hard if the owner is upset. Be gentle, but persistent enough to get all the information you need.

Common Small-Animal Emergencies

An emergency is any situation in which the pet seems in severe distress or discomfort. Some common small-animal emergencies are:

- Hit by a car or other trauma, such as a blow to

the head or some other part of the body

- A dog or cat in labor for more than one hour without puppies or kittens being born
- Severe vomiting and/or diarrhea
- Pet trying but unable to urinate
- Uncontrolled bleeding
- Heat stroke
- Severe dog or cat fight wounds
- Breathing difficulty; pet's tongue, gums turning blue
- Bloat
- Prolapsed eye
- Ingestion of antifreeze or other poison

Basic First Aid Advice for Clients

First muzzle the pet. Although a dog might never bite in normal circumstances, extreme pain can cause it to bite at almost anything, including its owner's hand. This advice should be given before all other instructions.

In cases of hemorrhage and uncontrolled bleeding, apply direct pressure or a pressure bandage at the site of the bleeding. Apply a clean, moist towel or rag on any wound, especially a prolapsed eye.

If there is a possibility of a back injury or a fracture—for example, when a pet has been hit by a car—advise the client to transport the pet on a stretcher. A piece of plywood works well.

Common Large-Animal Emergencies

Horses

Colic
Founder (laminitis)
Choke

Wounds/lacerations
Unable to foal (give birth)

Cattle

Calving (birthing) difficulties
Milk fever
Toxicities
Trauma/accidents
Choke

Swine

Farrowing (birthing) difficulties
Milk fever
Trauma/accidents

SUMMARY OF IMPORTANT POINTS

• Know your clinic's emergency plan and implement it as calmly and smoothly as possible when an emergency arises.

• If you're not sure if a problem is a true emergency, always treat it as if it is.

• Know your clinic's procedure for referring emergencies after hours or when the doctor is not available.

Notes

CHAPTER

8

Interacting With Clients

In Chapter 1 we discussed the importance of your attitude toward clients. A friendly smile and pleasant tone of voice make clients glad they decided to come to your clinic.

Another important aspect of your interaction with clients is accurate communication. This includes carefully listening to what the client is asking you to do for the pet as well as being clear in giving the client instructions. It includes being comforting and compassionate in times of grief and level-headed in times of anger or upset. As we'll see later, miscommunication can lead to misunderstandings and unhappy clients—something you definitely want to avoid!

Getting All the Details From the Client

When an animal comes in for treatment, confirm the purpose of the pet's visit. This information should be in the appointment book, but confirm it anyway. An owner will often think of something else to discuss with the doctor after the appointment has been made.

If there are no other concerns, ask if there is anything else the doctor can do while the pet is there. Check the chart to make sure all vaccinations and parasite checks are current. If the pet has had a continuing ailment, such as an allergy, ask the owner if the doctor should check it.

List everything the client has requested on the patient chart or a drop-off form. If the pet is staying at the hospital, get a phone number where the owner can be reached during the day, and be sure the pet is properly identified with a cage card and/or identification collar.

☛ TIP

Enter the animal on the day's treatment schedule immediately, or ask one of the technicians to do it. Always be sure that someone besides you knows the animal has been admitted to the hospital. No animal's treatment should be accidentally overlooked because no one knew it was there.

Giving Information to the Client

Soothing the Anxious Owner

Pet owners are often anxious, even fearful, about leaving their pets with the veterinarian. This is only natural. In many cases, owners do not have a clear understanding of the procedures their pets will undergo, yet they must entrust their pets to your clinic for care and treatment.

When you face an anxious owner, be sympathetic but in control. Reassure the client by saying, "I understand how you feel. We will take good care of Pooch, and you can call us at (name a specific time) to check on him." Or if the owner is *very* anxious, you might say, "I will call you the moment the doctor finishes the surgery." Then remove the pet to the kennel room or have an aide do so.

Confirm Discharge Time

Ideally, each client should be given a discharge appointment at the time the pet is left for treatment or surgery. Discharge appointments allow the doctor to speak with each client individually at the time of release and help prevent a crowd of people wanting to pick up their pets at exactly the same time at the end of the day.

When it is uncertain when the patient can go home, have the owner call to set up a discharge appointment.

Cost Estimates

Giving accurate estimates is the easiest way to avoid misunderstandings when you discharge a patient. Cost estimates should be made when the client makes the appointment, not when you are admitting the pet to the hospital. You will know the prices of your routine treatments and surgeries from your fee schedules and can give this information over the phone or print an estimate on the computer (see Chapter 5 on giving clients price information).

☛ TIP

When giving a client an estimate, whether verbal or printed, be sure he or she understands it is an estimate of the costs. Unforeseen circumstances, such as complications during surgery, may cause the final price to be different from the original estimate.

If you are not familiar with the surgery, ask the doctor to estimate the cost so you can call the client back with the estimate. If the procedure is expensive and the client has made arrangements with the doctor to pay in installments (see Chapter 5), make sure the terms of the payment plan are made clear *before* admitting the pet.

Settle the bill at the front desk before the pet is brought from the kennel room. This allows the client to pay without the distraction of a squirming pet and psychologically separates the payment from the pet. (See Chapter 5 for a more detailed discussion of settling the bill.)

Once payment is complete, escort the client to the exam room where the pet will be discharged. At this time, the client will receive special instructions from the doctor or, for routine cases, from the technician or you.

☛ TIP

Avoid discharging pets directly through the waiting room. It can lead to confusion and doesn't give the client your undivided attention during the release of the pet.

Remember your golden rule: Each client is special and deserves the best possible care for his or her pet.

Home-Care Instructions

As we have mentioned, the doctor sometimes will want to personally release certain cases. Charts for "doctor-release" patients should be clearly marked to be sure the pet has a discharge appointment and the doctor talks with the client.

If you will be releasing a pet, be sure you understand what to tell the client—either about the treatment the pet had at your clinic or what the owner must do at home.

Many clinics have preprinted home-care instructions for frequently performed surgeries and treatments. These instructions are useful but replace your personal touch! Go over the information with each owner, and point to or highlight specific parts of the instructions that pertain to the owner's pet. People are more likely to read and follow printed information if they have been shown why it is of particular interest to them.

Also, you must be sure the client understands the instructions. As you are talking with a client, don't be afraid to say, "Do you have any questions?" After all, in many cases, the home care can be just as important as the care the pet received at your hospital.

Grief Counseling

Death of a Pet

The death of a pet is a sad event. As a receptionist, you must learn to handle an animal's death sympathetically. At the same time, you must try not to become overly emotional. You don't want to further upset the client, and you need to take care of the details surrounding this unhappy event.

First, you will need to make burial arrangements for the pet. The owner may want to take care of burying the pet. If not, be sure you know what other options are available. Pet cemeteries offer burial and cremation services, and your local animal-control department may have a cremation facility or burial site. Familiarize yourself with the services in your area, and be ready to discuss them with the client.

Next, mark the pet's file "DECEASED" and remove it from the active files and from the computer. Remove all reminder cards from the file or computer. You don't want to renew the client's grief by sending vaccination reminders or inquiring about recently deceased pets.

If your doctor sends sympathy cards to owners of deceased pets, address an envelope for a personal note or card. Whether you or the doctor sends the card, *it should always be personally signed.*

Euthanasia

Perhaps the kindest thing an owner can do for a pet that is so sick or so severely injured that it will never recover normal health is to have the veterinarian induce its death quietly and humanely. This is called euthanasia.

The decision to have a pet euthanized is a serious one that is never easy to make. Occasionally you, as a receptionist, will have to deal with clients who choose to or must have a pet euthanized. In order for you to help grieving clients through a difficult time, you must understand what euthanasia is, how it is performed, and why there are certain cases when it is the kindest—perhaps the only—choice.

Euthanasia is the painless inducement of death, usually by intravenous injection, in a suffering animal. The decision to perform euthanasia is between the doctor and the client and depends on the nature of the pet's illness or the severity of its injury. Anxious owners may ask you if you think a pet will have to be put to sleep. Your best response is, "Euthanasia is a serious decision, and Dr. Jones would like to discuss it with you."

If the doctor and client decide that euthanasia is necessary, *be sure the client signs your hospital's euthanasia record or euthanasia permission form.* Your clinic may have preprinted slips for this purpose. Fill out the slip completely, and have the client sign it. Having clients sign such a form is often difficult because they are understandably upset at this time. Try to be understanding and sympathetic, but keep in mind that no pet may be euthanized until the form is signed.

The form serves several purposes. It is a record of the pet's death. It certifies that the animal has not bitten anyone or been exposed to rabies. It shows who had the pet euthanized. You will then follow the steps outlined above for making burial arrangements, purging or updating your files, and sending a sympathy card to the client.

☛ TIP

Discuss euthanasia with the doctor and other staff members ***before*** *you must discuss it with a client. Be sure you can talk about it without becoming overly emotional. While you never want to appear cold and uncaring with a client, you also don't want to break down in front of someone who is looking to you for strength and support.*

The Grieving Client

Some clients may find it difficult to adjust after the death of a pet. After all, the pet has been a close companion for years. Some clients may want to replace their pets right away. If so, you may be able to help them find a new dog or cat. Some people simply need time to go through the grieving process. If you have brochures or other literature about the death of a pet, you can offer them to the client. There are other sources of support, including:

Pet Loss Support Hotline, sponsored by the veterinary school at the University of California at Davis. Telephone: (800) 565-1526 or (530) 752-4200, from 6:30 p.m. to 9:30 p.m. Pacific Standard Time, Monday through Friday (Tuesday and Thursday during the summer.)

Grief counseling by Michigan State University veterinary student volunteers. Telephone: (517) 432-2696, from 7 p.m. to 9 p.m. Eastern Standard Time, Tuesday and Thursday.

American Animal Hospital Association Grief Brochure. Member Service Center, P.O. Box 150899, Denver, CO 80215. Telephone: (800) 252-2242 to request information. You can also request information via e-mail at AAHA@aol.com.

Two good books to help children deal with a pet's death are:

The Tenth Good Thing About Barney, by Judith Viorst (Aladdin Press) and

When a Pet Dies, by Fred Rogers, TV's *Mister Rogers* (G.P. Putnam's Sons).

In addition, many communities have local support groups to help grieving pet owners. A local pet cemetery may have information on such groups. Check what's available in your area and list them below:

Local Support Groups for Grieving Pet Owners

The Unhappy Client

Not everyone is happy all of the time. And occasionally there will be a client who marches into a full waiting room and targets you, the receptionist, as the person responsible. An unhappy client needs special attention.

If someone is shouting at you, your natural reaction might be to shout back or to leave the situation. As a veterinary receptionist, you can not do either of these. Most unhappy clients simply want to be heard—they want to get their grievances out in the open. It is your job to understand the client's problem and to help remedy it.

Just as you practiced for the emergencies that come into your clinic, you must practice communicating with an unhappy client. Role playing is valuable in learning what to say and how to say it.

Putting Out the Fire

There are four important steps in dealing with clients who are unhappy, angry, or upset:

1. Let the client know you realize he or she is upset.
2. Find out the reason why.
3. Work out a solution for the problem.
4. Record in your notebook ("Client Complaints/Problems") exactly what happened, and label the client folder as well.

We will deal with each of these steps in detail, but first let's clarify what we mean when we talk about an unhappy client.

What Makes a Client Unhappy?

Most clients who register complaints are either dissatisfied with their pet's treatment or unhappy about the cost of services. Dissatisfaction with the service itself is most often the result of one of the following:

1. The client's perception of an uncaring attitude on the part of the hospital staff.
2. Failure of the clinic staff to perform all the services the client wanted. This happens when the client has requested several services, and one (or more) is forgotten or omitted.
3. Failure to complete a service to the client's satisfaction. For example, a pet might go home dirty after a bath or still have fleas after it has been dipped.
4. Unwanted results of a service. For example, surgery to repair a broken bone was successful, but the patient had an allergic reaction to the rabies vaccine and died.

A client's dissatisfaction with the cost of service usually results from:

1. Quoting one cost and charging another. As we said earlier, this dissatisfaction is best avoided through good communication. An estimate and a current running balance for hospitalized patients go a long way toward preventing this problem.
2. Failure of the client to perceive the value of the services rendered. (See Chapter 5 for ways to prevent this.)

"I Understand"

Let's look at a client complaint and work through each of our four steps to resolve the problem.

Mrs. Smith is at your door when the clinic opens in the morning. She says to you, "I paid you people $18 yesterday, and just look at Sparky today! Why, he's no better off now than yesterday morning. Neither one of us got any sleep last night. You people are going to have to do better than this if you expect us to keep coming here!"

Don't freeze up! Don't get angry! This client has a problem, and you must get your mind set to help her solve it. *Put yourself in a communicating mood.*

Your first response is to acknowledge the client's unhappiness. *Let the client know you realize she is upset!*

You do this by saying, "Mrs. Smith, I can see you're really upset about this, and I want to resolve this problem. It's upsetting for us when we have an unhappy client. It's our job to provide the best possible service for each pet and to make each owner happy. Let's figure out the best way to resolve this situation."

Now is the time to remove the client to a comfortable area, one which is private and has no audience to fuel the client's fire by creating a feeling that she is "performing." An office or an empty exam room is ideal. Remember, your job is to maintain a pleasant atmosphere in the front office, and you can't do that when someone is upset. So, just as you removed the emergency victim and its owner, you must remove the unhappy client from the waiting room by saying, "You seem to be upset, and I want to understand and help you with this problem, Mrs. Smith. Please come to the exam room with me so we can discuss it and you can give me all the details."

"Why Are You Upset?"

You have just told Mrs. Smith that you want to know why she is unhappy. Now is the time to listen to the problem—*all of it*—even to the point of taking notes. You might begin by saying, "I'm sorry you're so upset, Mrs. Smith." Try to recognize what the client feels, and encourage her to tell you exactly why she is unhappy.

"Well, yesterday I left Sparky here all day for a bath and dip. I wanted to pick him up at 2 o'clock, but you said he had to stay all day. And when I finally took him home last night, he *still* had fleas and he scratched all night long. I think that for $18 you should have done a better job."

Recognize how the client feels: "I'm glad I understand the situation now, Mrs. Smith. If I were you, I would be upset, too. You brought Sparky here to get rid of his fleas, and he still has fleas. I think we can resolve this problem."

"What Can We Do to Resolve the Problem?"

In the above example, the obvious resolution is to rebathe and redip Sparky at no charge to Mrs. Smith, and to discuss monthly flea control products and home treatment products to help her avoid this problem in the future. In other situations you may want to ask the client, "How would you like to see this situation resolved? We want you to be happy and would like to have your suggestions for solving this problem."

☛ TIP

Remember, it's not only what you say but how you say it. Your tone of voice and body language convey more meaning than your actual words. Be careful how you speak!

Take Notes!

As we discussed in Chapter 2, you should have a notebook in which you keep track of client complaints. You should enter in your notebook any client complaint or problem, along with how you resolved the situation. For example: "8/8/00: Mrs. Smith's dog Sparky was bathed and dipped here yesterday. She brought Sparky back this morning because he still had fleas. Resolution: Sparky was bathed and dipped again at no charge. Discussed a monthly flea control and home foggers." Once you have logged this in your notebook, put a note on Mrs. Smith's chart that this problem occurred and how it was resolved. After all, you never want to make the same mistake twice.

When to Call the Doctor

Through reflective listening ("I'm sorry you're upset") and sympathizing ("I understand") you will be able to resolve most client problems. But occasionally there will be a situation that you feel is beyond your powers of reasoning or out of your control. When this happens, remember:

The ultimate goal in dealing with an unhappy person is to retain that person as a client.

If you feel the doctor has a better chance of resolving the problem and keeping the client, then get the doctor involved. Take time, however, to brief the doctor fully before bringing in the client.

If the client uses abusive language or yells at you, do not resort to the same level of communication. Quietly tell the client, "As soon as you calm down, I or the doctor will be glad to talk to you about why you are upset." If the client continues to be abusive, say, "I can see that you are too upset to talk about this right now. I will be back when we can discuss this calmly." Then leave the room, and alert the doctor to the situation.

When the Unhappy Client Is on the Phone

You may feel at a slight disadvantage when you are trying to communicate with an unhappy client on the phone. It's always easier when you are face to face. But you should handle a caller the same way you would someone in the waiting room. Be communicative and understanding. Follow the steps to identify the problem and to resolve it.

If you feel that you and the client are not communicating well, invite the client to come to the office to discuss the problem. For example, "Mr. Brown, I want to understand and help you with this problem. Could you come to the office so we can put our heads together and resolve this situation?"

An Ounce of Prevention . . .

Of course, the easiest way to deal with client problems is to prevent them. Study the lists at the beginning of this section that describe why clients become unhappy clients. Go over each point, and ask yourself, "What can we do to prevent this from happening in our clinic?" This is an excellent topic for a staff meeting, with members of each department contributing ways to increase efficiency and cut down on problems.

For example, you might say, "When a client comes in with a long list of services, I will write down each service, read the list back, and be sure that I have everything noted on the pet's chart."

A kennel worker might say, "I will double-check every pet that's had a bath and dip to be sure it doesn't have any fleas when it goes home."

The better the communication among the staff members, the better you will serve your clients!

➤ POINT TO PONDER

The unhappy client is doing you a favor by complaining. Rather than going to another clinic, the client is giving you a reason for the dissatisfaction and a chance to improve your services. Always listen to client complaints carefully and treat them seriously. You can often turn a bad situation into a valuable learning experience.

SUMMARY OF IMPORTANT POINTS

• Always convey a caring attitude toward clients and toward their pets.

• Communicate clearly. Be sure you understand the client and that the client understands you.

• If a client has a problem, *listen* to the client and take steps to resolve the problem to the client's satisfaction.

Notes

CHAPTER

9

Your Role in Marketing

You are the most important marketing tool your clinic has. Wait a minute, you might say. I never went to business school. I'm a veterinary receptionist. What do I know about marketing?

More than you think! According to marketing expert Philip Kotler, marketing is nothing more than satisfying the needs and wants of your customers through exchange processes.

This means that you try to find out what your clients want and do your best to provide it for them. You even try to figure out what they want *before* they ask you for it. Anticipate their needs and satisfy their wants. In doing this, you help attract new clients and help your practice grow.

You deal with clients on a daily basis and project your clinic's image. In day-to-day business, you market your clinic best by being friendly to the clients, sympathetic to their problems, knowledgeable enough to answer their questions, and caring toward their pets. Every time you smile, listen attentively, or act efficiently, you help promote your clinic.

But there are other ways that you, as a receptionist, can help your practice grow and attract new clients. As you read through the following suggestions, ask yourself, "Am I doing this now? Is this something I could be more conscientious about? Would the doctor want me to do this?"

In addition to going over the marketing tips in this chapter, you may want to read the American Veterinary Medical Association's *Marketing and Practice Strategies for the Companion Animal Practice* for more useful information. Also, you and your doctor may come up with a list of your own marketing tips. Add your tips to those listed here. It will help you remember to put them into practice and will be a good aid for you in training new receptionists.

Call-Backs and Rechecks

Generate a recall list for all patients who have had surgery in your clinic. You can save a lot of time by letting your computer do the legwork—many software programs allow you to link a recall to a specific piece of surgery or you can enter it manually—or you can use a notebook devoted to recalls.

The day after a pet's surgery, call the client and say, "Dr. Jones wanted to know how Spunky was feeling after his surgery." If the surgery requires removal of stitches, set a new recall date to make an appointment for suture removal or schedule the appointment while you have the client on the phone.

If time permits in your clinic, add sick pets, pets suffering from allergies, and pets treated for non-routine ailments to your recall list. You project a caring image for your clinic when you follow up with clients on the treatment their pets received. It also allows you to schedule recheck appointments for pets whose recovery is not as rapid as it should be or pets whose progress must be monitored by the doctor.

Reminders

Be conscientious about your reminder system. Be sure your vaccination reminders are mailed out on time, and carefully look through your files for clients whose pets are past due on their vaccinations. Call these people to schedule appointments. A good approach on the telephone is, "Mrs. Smith, I sent you a postcard last month and was afraid you might not have received it. Because Spot is a little past due on his yearly vaccinations, I was wondering if you'd like to make an appointment to get that done."

Lost Pets

You will receive many phone calls from people who have lost their pets. Always record the caller's name, address, and phone number, as well as a description of the pet and call the person back in a few days to see if the pet has been found. Do this even if the caller is not a regular client. When the pet is found or replaced, the owner may remember that you cared enough to call back and may choose your clinic for the pet's veterinary needs.

Your clinic may want to provide clients with "lost pet kits" that provide pet photos, which can be taken at the clinic with an instant camera, and a vendor source list for identification tags. Be sure to also include safety tips and ways to prevent pets from becoming lost.

Many veterinarians now implant microchips under the skin of dogs and cats. These microchips can be read by scanners at animal shelters and compared against a nationwide register. Check with the doctor to see if this can be done in conjunction with other routine surgery, such as spaying or neutering, at little or no cost to the client.

Price Shoppers

Price shoppers are important to your clinic. When someone calls you to ask the price of a procedure, you learn that the caller owns a pet, is not affiliated with another veterinarian, is willing to spend money on the pet, and is a potential client.

Your goal is to make an appointment for the price shopper—allowing the doctor to examine the pet and (we hope!) convert the owner into a regular client.

Even if you don't succeed in making an appointment, try to get the caller's name and address so you can mail a clinic brochure and information on the procedure inquired about. Attach a note saying: "Thank you for calling our clinic. I hope we can help you in the future. Enclosed is some information about us and about the procedure you were interested in. If you have any other questions, please give us a call." You may want to print these notecards on your computer or have them preprinted.

Referrals

There should be a question on your new client-information sheet or registration form that asks, "Whom may we thank for sending you to us?" If the client leaves it blank, ask how the clinic was chosen. Doing so helps the doctor to know whether new business is coming from the yellow pages, the sign outside, or other clients. Keep track of clients who refer new people to your office. A client who sends a friend or neighbor to your clinic has paid you a big compliment and should be thanked. A typical thank-you note might read as follows:

Referral Thank-You Note

Dear Mrs. Lawson,

Thank you for sending Paula Brown and Sassy to our clinic. We appreciate your confidence in us.

Have the doctor sign each card personally or sign, "The doctors and staff at Main Street Animal Clinic."

If you keep track of your referrals and find that a

particular client is sending you several every month, do something special for that client—send a rosebud with a note saying, "Thanks for all the new people you have sent to our clinic. We sincerely appreciate your confidence in us." A small gift at Christmas or Thanksgiving might also be appropriate.

New Clients

Just as you thank clients for referrals, you should also welcome new clients to the practice. You may want to have some preprinted cards on hand for this, but be sure the doctor signs each card personally. Let the clients know that you care about them and their pets!

Hand out clinic brochures and business cards to all new clients and to clients who haven't been in for a while. It's also a good idea to have seasonal literature on hand to give to new clients—for example, flea control in the summer, heartworm prevention in the spring, winterizing pets in the fall, and Christmas puppies in the winter. No new client should leave your clinic without several items that include the clinic name. Use every opportunity available to remind current and potential clients that your clinic provides not only the best care for their pets but offers useful and timely information as well.

Deceased Pets

Having a pet die is a traumatic experience. Ask your doctor if you should send sympathy cards to clients whose pets have died. Many clinics have these cards preprinted and then write a personal note on the card as well. Like the other mailings, be sure to sign sympathy cards personally. Other doctors may want to make a donation to a foundation in the name of the deceased pet. For example, if the pet died of cancer, a donation would go to a veterinary cancer foundation.

NOTE: The moment you learn of the death of a pet, remove the pet and all vaccination reminders pertaining to that pet from your computer and files. It is very painful to the owner to receive a reminder for a pet who is gone and embarrassing for you when you inquire about the health of a pet who died several months ago.

Some clinics have a large erasable board that lists all recently deceased pets to help staff members remember who has died. This helps prevent the slip-ups mentioned above. Naturally, such a board would be kept out of view of clients and might be titled "In Memory Of" in case a client should see it.

New Product Education

When you start dispensing a new over-the-counter product, be sure that you understand its purpose and can give clear instructions for its use. The doctor may train you in this area or have a sales representative from the product's company instruct you in its uses and benefits.

☛ TIP

Use preprinted labels or a rubber stamp to mark all products with your clinic's name, address, and phone number. Clients will be more likely to return to your clinic when they run out of the product.

Product Follow-up

Keep track of the over-the-counter products that your clients buy, either by using your computer or recording the purchase in the clients' files. That will enable you to follow up with clients by asking, for example, how the pet likes the new food or if the medicated shampoo helped clear up a rash. It's another way to show how much you care about your clients' pets.

First Exam Follow-up

As a new client leaves your office after a first visit, it's a good idea to have a short exit interview. Ask the client if there are any questions about the pet's exam, the doctor's instructions, or hospital policy. If the doctor recommended follow-up treatment, ask if an appointment could be made at that time. And always ask if there is anything else you can do for the client.

Client Needs

Are you being asked the same question over and over lately? Has the same product been requested 10 times in the last two weeks? Be alert to the needs of your clients. For example, if you notice that you get many questions every day about flea and tick control, suggest to the doctor that he or she write an article for the local paper outlining the problem and its solution. You could also prepare a handout on the subject and make it available to all your clients. If a certain product is requested frequently, mention it to the doctor or do some research on the product and present your findings to the doctor.

The Waiting Room

Your waiting room should be as neat and comfortable as your living room. Make it a practice to enter the clinic through the waiting room every day. Look at it as if you had never seen it before. Be critical. Is the floor clean and free of hair? Is the seating clean and neat? Are the magazines and other reading material arranged neatly?

Give your waiting room the sniff test. Are there any offensive odors? Do this when you first enter because after you've been at work for a while you'll no longer notice unpleasant odors.

Employee Photo Album

Clients are almost always interested in the clinic employees and their pets. Have the employees (and the doctors, too!) bring in a few photos of themselves at home with their pets. Arrange them in an album with employee and pet names labeled, and leave the album in the waiting room for clients. They enjoy looking at the pictures and can see that everyone at the clinic likes animals and enjoys their own pets. This helps your clients feel confident they are entrusting the care of their pets to a staff that truly takes pride in providing the best possible care for the animals in their charge.

Hospital Photo Album

Another album you might want to put together is one of the various departments at your clinic, showing the employees at work. Many clients wonder what goes on in the treatment room or the laboratory. Label each picture with the name of the department and the employee who works there. Give a brief description of the department and the job.

Client Photo Album

Ask your clients for pictures of their pets, and put them in an album with names and dates labeled. Note interesting things about the pets or that they were good patients when they stayed at your clinic.

Take a picture each time a client brings a new pet in for an appointment and post the picture on a bulletin board in the reception area.

Making the Most of Your Computer

Your computer can provide you with a lot of information that will help you market your clinic. In addition to keeping up with past-due reminders, your computer can target certain patients for the selective mailing of letters, brochures, and other information.

For example, each month you might want to ask your computer to give you the names of all the pets that have just turned 6 months old. You could then send a letter to each owner, describing the benefits of spaying, neutering, dental checks, heartworm checks, and parvovirus boosters.

Other topics for patient selection might include older pets; dogs that have been treated for heartworms; and pets with chronic problems, such as allergies, ear problems, gum disease, or other ailments.

Your computer will also enable you to send a quarterly newsletter to your clients. A newsletter should be short—one page, perhaps—and might address a seasonal problem. One important point about newsletters: Once you start sending them, don't stop. People get used to receiving something from you in the mail and may wonder if you're still in business if the newsletters stop coming!

E-Mail Opportunities

Through e-mail, you can alert clients about seasonal topics—just as you would in a printed newsletter—and answer questions for busy clients who find it hard to call during normal business hours. One word of caution: Answering e-mail can be a time consuming business. If you don't have the time to answer every single e-mail that comes in, don't offer this option for your clients! Queries from clients should never go ignored.

You might want to revise your new-client information sheet to ask, "Would you like to receive information about topics important to your pet's health via e-mail? If so, please include your e-mail address here." Then once a month—or whatever schedule the doctor sets—you can send a short electronic newsletter to those clients. Just as with the printed newsletter, once you start sending it, don't stop—or your clients will wonder why.

Clinic Web Site

Some clinics are going online as a way of providing information to their clients. Ideally, a clinic's Web site would cover the same material that's in your clinic brochure: name and address of the clinic (along with the exact location), clinic phone numbers and hours, types of animals treated, any specialties, and short biographies and credentials of the doctors who practice there.

If creating a Web site seems overwhelming, don't panic. There's plenty of help out there. Local college computer departments and computer companies can often help. Chances are one of your clients knows how to develop a Web site. You can find help online from the American Animal Hospital Association, at www.aahanet.org. There you'll find links to sample Web pages.

Other sites provide templates for developing Web pages. Use one of the many search engines and type in "Web design." Yale University, for example, has a helpful site at http://info.med.yale.edu/caim/manual/contents.html.

If you decide to develop a Web page, be sure you keep it current. Update seasonal tips regularly and post changes in personnel, hours, or types of animals treated as soon as possible.

SUMMARY OF IMPORTANT POINTS

- Maintain a friendly, caring attitude.
- Keep clients' needs in mind at all times. Try to anticipate these needs so you can meet them easily.
- Add a personal touch to client interactions whenever possible. Stay in touch with phone calls, mailings, and e-mail.

Notes

CHAPTER

10

The Importance of Diagnostic Tests

An accurate diagnosis of an animal's illness is based on several different types of information. A doctor's diagnosis usually begins by asking the owner to give a history of the problem:

1. What is the nature of the problem?
2. When did the problem start?
3. In a herd of animals, how many are affected?
4. What, if anything, has been done?

Next the doctor performs a complete physical examination, taking the animal's temperature, weighing it, and examining it from head to toe. If an animal is in pain, the physical exam will often pinpoint the painful area.

However, not every illness can be diagnosed through a physical examination. Various diagnostic aids help the doctor by providing more information about the animal's condition. These include laboratory tests, radiology (X-ray), electrocardiography (ECG), electroencephalography (EEG), ultrasonography, endoscopy, and computer-enhanced images. Let's look at some of these.

Laboratory Tests

Just as the physical exam tells the doctor about the external condition of the animal, laboratory tests give information about the internal condition. Lab tests can be performed on almost anything—food, water, bodily fluids, feces, blood, urine, or tissues. Many lab tests can be done in the veterinary hospital, but the more complex tests may be performed by outside laboratories.

The following list describes some of the most commonly performed "in-house" lab tests.

Blood Tests

ALT (SGPT)—determines liver function.

AST (SGOT)—determines liver/muscle function.

Bilirubin—determines liver function.

BUN—determines kidney function.

Clotting Time—determines blood-clotting function.

Complete Blood Count (CBC)—determines the total count of all types of blood cells, which helps detect infection or other abnormalities.

Creatinine—determines kidney function.

Electrolytes—determines sodium and potassium levels; imbalances of these can be life-threatening.

Glucose—helps diagnose diabetes.

Hematocrit or Packed Cell Volume (PCV)—determines the percentage of red blood cells in the blood; this helps to detect anemia.

Thyroid Function—determines if thyroid gland function is normal, elevated, or decreased.

Other Tests

Ear Swab—detects yeast, bacteria, or mites in the ear.

Fecal Flotation—detects intestinal parasites by examining stool sample under the microscope.

FeLV/FIV—blood test that indicates the presence of feline leukemia virus and feline immunodeficiency virus in cats.

FIP—detects the presence of feline infectious peritonitis in cats.

Fungal Culture—detects the presence of ringworm and other fungal infections.

Heartworm Test—several types of heartworm tests are available. Some types detect microfilariae (juvenile heartworms) and other types detect proteins from adult heartworms or proteins produced by the pet in response to heartworm infection.

Needle Aspirate—a "minibiopsy" performed on a small number of tissue cells obtained with a needle.

Skin Scraping—microscopic examination of skin cells to detect the presence of mange mites.

Skin Swab—swab taken from skin, then rolled on a microscope slide and stained in order to identify bacteria and yeast.

Urinalysis—indicates kidney function; often detects urinary tract infection.

Vaginal Swab—determines the stage of the heat cycle and time of ovulation. Often used in dogs and horses for breeding purposes.

Outside Lab Tests

In Chapter 2, we discussed ways to keep track of outside lab tests. Usually a clinic uses only one or two outside labs, and each lab should provide you with a complete list of the tests it performs. Keep all of your outside lab information, along with your own lab logbook, in one spot at the front desk. This way, when the doctor tells you to have a certain test run at a certain lab, you'll know exactly where to look to find the necessary information.

When the lab calls you with the results of a test, record them on a form provided by the lab. Some labs will fax results, eliminating the need to take results over the phone.

Notify the doctor of test results as soon as they are available. The doctor will inform the owner of the results and decide on a course of treatment.

Radiology

Another diagnostic tool is the radiograph, or X-ray—the picture the doctor takes to diagnose broken bones, dislocations, and other internal problems that cannot be seen during an external examination.

As the name implies, an X-ray machine generates special radiation to penetrate tissue and create a picture that lets the doctor "see inside" an animal without surgery.

Radiology can also be helpful in diagnosing heart disease (with a picture of an enlarged heart), urinary tract problems (by revealing bladder stones), and cancer (with a picture of a large mass or tumor), as well as in locating foreign bodies (when a cat has swallowed a needle or a dog has been shot).

Ultrasonography

Like the X-ray, ultrasonography gives an internal picture. It is a sonar device that monitors the reflection of sound waves it sends out and creates an image of what it "sees" on a video screen. These sophisticated machines have a wide variety of uses. They can create images of internal organs and are useful in detecting early pregnancies, heart problems, and tumors.

Endoscopy

The endoscope is a semiflexible tool with a fiberoptic light source. It allows the doctor to see whatever is at the end of the tube. For example, when it is inserted into the esophagus, the doctor can see directly into the stomach. Instead of having to look at an image as with X-ray and ultrasound, the doctor gets a firsthand look inside an animal without performing surgery. An endoscope is especially useful to treat horses. Doctors use it to look into airways, sinuses, the esophagus, and the stomach. It is also commonly used for gastrointestinal, airway, and bladder problems in dogs and cats.

Computer-Enhanced Images

These noninvasive tests are becoming more available in veterinary medicine. Computed tomography (CT scan or CAT scan) and magnetic resonance imaging (MRI) use computers to collect and process information into a model of the area. The main difference between the two: CT scan uses X-ray and is good for bony areas, and MRI uses magnetic fields and is excellent for soft tissue areas. For example, a CT scan is commonly used for nasal tumors, brain tumors, and bone and joint problems. The MRI is often used for central nervous system imaging for tumors, disc problems, and ligament damage.

Notes

CHAPTER

11

The Importance of Vaccinations

What Is a Vaccination?

A vaccination, or immunization, is medicine's way of helping an animal to protect itself against disease. This is called preventive medicine—you prevent the disease before it happens. A good program of preventive medicine is every veterinarian's goal. When you vaccinate an animal, you make it immune, or resistant, to certain diseases. Most vaccines are injected into the body, but some are given orally or intranasally. A vaccine is a specific protein that stimulates the body to produce antibodies against a disease. These antibodies create an *active immunity.*

Newborns acquire a *passive immunity* from their mothers, who pass on antibodies to the newborn through nursing or from inside the uterus. This prevents newborns from catching contagious diseases as soon as they are born.

Why Do Animals Need Vaccinations?

Because a young animal's passive immunity is temporary, veterinarians must help it keep up its resistance to disease. Therefore, they vaccinate it to protect it. Immunizations begin at an early age and are given in a series to ensure good protection. *The young animal is not immune until it has completed the entire series of vaccinations.*

Unless indicated otherwise, all the vaccines discussed in this chapter require an initial series of two to four vaccinations, followed by regular boosters.

Dog Diseases and Vaccination Schedules

The dog, or canine, vaccination series usually begins when puppies are 6 to 8 weeks old. The series consists of three or four visits, the last of which takes place when the puppy is about 4 months old. Once the puppy has completed the "puppy shots," it should return to the veterinarian for booster vaccinations to maintain a protective antibody level. Veterinarians commonly vaccinate dogs for:

Canine Distemper

A highly contagious disease caused by a virus. It is spread among dogs by contact through the mouth or nose. The virus can attack all parts of the body, including the nervous system. It is usually fatal.

Hepatitis

A viral infection of the liver. It is specific to the canine family—that means that this particular virus is not contagious to humans. Canine hepatitis virus is sometimes referred to as canine adenovirus type 1. Hepatitis is transmitted when dogs ingest the virus in contaminated water and may be fatal.

Kennel Cough

An infection caused by the *Bordetella* bacterium and the parainfluenza virus. The disease, also known as infectious tracheobronchitis, is characterized by a continual honking bronchial cough. It is transmitted when an infected dog coughs and infective particles are inhaled by other dogs. As the name implies, it can be easily transmitted in a kennel where many dogs are present.

Leptospirosis

A bacterial infection spread through water contaminated with infected urine. It is more common in rural areas and is marked by a high fever and yellow or icteric-colored gums. It can cause permanent kidney damage and can be fatal if untreated.

Lyme Disease

A disease that infects the musculoskeletal system, heart, and kidneys. Lyme disease—named for the town of Lyme, Conn., where the disease was first reported in humans—is caused by the *Borrelia* organism and is transmitted by *Ixodes* tick bites. In areas where ticks are prevalent, doctors may vaccinate for Lyme disease annually.

Parvovirus and Coronavirus Infections

Infections of the dog's intestinal tract. A parvovirus infection is usually more severe than a coronavirus infection—in fact it is often fatal. The parvovirus and coronavirus cause severe vomiting and diarrhea. The diarrhea is usually bloody and has a very foul odor. Both diseases are transmitted by viral particles (found in feces) that are inhaled through the nose or the mouth.

Rabies

Transmitted by the rabies virus, which enters the body through a break in the skin—often a bite from an infected animal. It is almost always fatal. Rabies is contagious to *all* land mammals, including humans. It is a very serious disease and should never be taken lightly. That's why there's so much emphasis on rabies vaccinations. It's important for owners to get their pets immunized and keep their vaccinations current. In fact, in most states the law requires that dogs and cats be current on their rabies vaccinations.

NOTE: There currently is no rabies vaccine licensed for use in wild animals. Wild animals, especially raccoons and skunks, often carry the virus without showing signs of the disease. Most veterinarians don't recommend keeping wild animals as pets.

Cat Diseases and Vaccination Schedules

The cat, or feline, vaccination series also begins when kittens are 6 to 8 weeks of age. The cat series consists of two or three visits. Like the dog, the cat needs boosters to maintain a good level of protective antibodies. The feline diseases that veterinarians have vaccines for include the following.

Feline Distemper

A viral disease that causes severe intestinal upset, vomiting, and diarrhea. It is highly contagious among cats and is transmitted by contact with the distemper virus through the cat's mouth or nose. Feline distemper is a serious disease and often fatal.

NOTE: Feline distemper is not the same as canine distemper. Distemper is not contagious between dogs and cats.

Feline Infectious Peritonitis (FIP)

Another leading viral killer of cats, second only to feline leukemia. FIP has two forms—wet and dry. Clinical signs of the wet form include fluid in the abdomen, fluid in the chest, and a persistent fever. The dry form can be difficult to diagnose, as some of the telltale signs often do not appear. FIP is fatal after clinical signs develop. The vaccine for FIP is intranasal—it is squirted into the nose rather than injected with a needle.

Feline Leukemia

This viral disease is the leading viral killer among cats and is transmitted from cat to cat by direct contact. The feline leukemia virus may cause leukemia or just an elevated temperature of unknown origin. It also may cause cancerous growths or anemia, which is a lack of red blood cell production. Support and treatment of an infected cat is costly, and the disease is usually fatal.

NOTE: At present, there have been no conclusive studies that show a cross-infection of the feline leukemia virus between cats and humans.

Rabies

See discussion on canine rabies.

Upper Respiratory Diseases

A disease complex that has three main causes: the rhinotracheitis virus (a herpesvirus), the calicivirus, and the chlamydia bacteria. Protection against all of these is available in one vaccine. A cat with an upper respiratory disease acts like a human with a cold. Clinical signs include sneezing, runny eyes, and difficulty breathing. It is highly contagious and transmitted from cat to cat by inhaling infective particles through the nose and mouth.

Horse Diseases and Vaccination Schedules

The horse, or equine, vaccinations begin early in life. In fact, foals should be vaccinated for tetanus at birth. Like puppies and kittens, young horses must have a series of vaccinations at a young age in order to be fully immunized. After the initial series, annual boosters are recommended. Veterinarians commonly vaccinate horses for the following diseases:

Encephalomyelitis

A viral disease that attacks the nervous system. Also called sleeping sickness, clinical signs include severe dullness or depression, inability to swallow, sleeping for abnormally long periods of time, uncoordinated gait, high fever, and partial loss of vision. Even if the horse survives the disease, the neurological damage is often permanent. There are two common strains of this disease: eastern and western. Both strains are prevalent throughout the United States, and vaccination for both is vital.

Equine Influenza (Flu)

A viral disease much like flu in humans. Clinical signs include coughing, nasal discharge, appetite loss, fever, and depression. The virus is airborne and is easily transmitted from horse to horse. Regular vaccination for show and performance horses is highly recommended.

Equine Rhinopneumonitis

A viral disease with two different forms. The respiratory form produces a severe infection in the upper respiratory tract. The horse will be very congested and will have trouble breathing. Because this form is highly contagious, yearly vaccination is recommended after the initial series. Many show and performance animals that are constantly exposed to other horses are vaccinated as frequently as four times a year. The uterine form of rhinopneumonitis infects the uterus of the pregnant mare and can cause a mare to abort her foal before it comes to full term. Many veterinarians vaccinate pregnant mares for rhinopneumonitis during the fifth, seventh, and ninth months of gestation.

Strangles

A disease caused by the *Streptococcus equi* bacterium. It primarily infects the upper respiratory tract and can cause abscesses in the throat. Transmitted by contaminated objects and by direct contact, strangles is a very dangerous disease. Doctors may recommend regular vaccinations, depending on the prevalence of strangles in your area.

NOTE: There are other equine diseases that may be important in certain areas of the country or in special situations. These include rabies, equine viral arteritis, and Potomac horse fever. Check with your doctor for specific vaccination recommendations on other equine diseases.

Tetanus

A disease caused by the tetanus bacterium *Clostridium tetani.* The organism enters the horse's body through a cut or puncture wound. Once inside the body it produces a poison, or a toxin. The toxin can cause respiratory paralysis and muscular rigidity, especially of the muscles in the neck and jaw area. This is why the condition is called lockjaw in humans. The disease is usually fatal, and regular tetanus toxoid vaccinations are a must for horses.

NOTE: There are two types of tetanus vaccine. *Tetanus antitoxin* gives a horse immediate, but temporary, protection against tetanus. The protection lasts about 10 days. It is given to newborn foals and to horses that have suffered puncture or other wounds but have never been vaccinated for tetanus. The *tetanus toxoid* vaccine, on the other hand, provides lasting immunity, but it doesn't take effect as quickly as the antitoxin.

Your Hospital's Immunization Schedules

Although all doctors basically give the same immunizations, some group them differently or space them out in various ways. It is important that you learn how these vaccinations are scheduled at your hospital.

Use the chart on the following page to outline your vaccination policies for dogs, cats, and horses.

Vaccination Updates

The veterinary healthcare industry is constantly seeking to upgrade the quality of patient care. Our vaccines have improved tremendously in the ability to stimulate protective titers. Because of these long-lasting titers, the advantages of vaccinations must be weighed against the small possibility of inducing tumors in cats and immune mediated diseases in dogs. Vaccines and protocols are constantly being studied and revised. Check with your doctor regarding the latest updates and protocols.

Notes

Summary of Vaccinations					
	Age at				
	1st shot	2nd	3rd	4th	Booster
Canine					
Distemper					
Hepatitis					
Leptospirosis					
Parainfluenza					
Parvovirus					
Coronavirus					
Kennel cough					
Rabies					
Lyme disease					
Other					
Feline					
Rhinotracheitis					
Calicivirus					
Panleukopenia					
FIP					
Leukemia					
Rabies					
Other					
Equine					
Tetanus					
Rhinopneumonitis					
Encephalomyelitis					
Influenza					
Strangles					
Other					

CHAPTER

12

The Importance of Internal Parasite Control

What Is a Parasite?

A parasite is an organism that lives at the expense of another living being. Internal parasites, such as intestinal worms and heartworms, live inside the body. Dogs, cats, and horses are subject to a variety of internal parasites, but some parasites are species-specific. In this chapter we will look at what you need to know about common internal parasites.

Dog and Cat Parasites

Coccidia

Coccidia are small protozoan parasites rather than worms. They are seen primarily in young animals, particularly those pets involved in stressful situations—such as moving to a new home. The coccidia cause irritation and inflammation of the intestine, which leads to diarrhea. Transmitted mainly by direct contact with other animals, coccidiosis is treated with oral medication. Treatment with oral medication is normally very effective.

Hookworms

Description: Hookworms are a very serious parasite problem, especially in young animals. The hookworm attaches itself to the intestinal wall and ingests blood. When left untreated, hookworms can cause "hookworm anemia," which is often fatal. Paleness of the gums and tongue and a black, tarry stool are the main signs of hookworm infestation.

The hookworm larvae can penetrate the skin to infect its host. *This includes humans!* Great care should be taken when cleaning an area infected by hookworms. Always wear gloves, and never walk barefoot or allow children to play in or around the infected area.

Treatment: Because hookworm eggs pass out in the stool, they can be detected by a fecal flotation test. If hookworms are present, the doctor gives the animal worm medication. Infected pets should be rechecked and/or dewormed again in several weeks.

Prevention: Prevention is similar for hookworms and roundworms. Keeping the yard clean and free of stools and checking the animal for worms at an early age will help prevent infestation. Sprays that kill hookworm larvae are available for yard infestation, and oral medication taken daily or monthly is available to control hookworms.

Roundworms

Description: Adult roundworms attach to the wall of the intestine and drain protein from the host. For this reason, roundworms are most harmful to young animals, which need as much nourishment as possible while they're growing.

Humans also can be infected by roundworms. If roundworm eggs are ingested by a human, the roundworm larvae can migrate throughout the body, causing a condition called visceral larval migrans. Children should never be allowed to play in areas contaminated by roundworm eggs.

Treatment: Roundworm eggs can be detected under the microscope by a fecal flotation test (see Chapter 10). Because roundworm eggs indicate the presence of adult roundworms, the doctor administers a worm medicine. Animals that are severely infested should be rechecked and/or dewormed again several weeks after the initial diagnosis.

Prevention: Early detection is important. When infestation occurs, owners must pick up all stool in the yard regularly. An oral medication, taken daily or monthly, is available for control of roundworms.

Clinic Policies on Intestinal Parasites

Age to first check puppies/kittens for worms: ______

When to check breeding females: ________________

When to check pregnant females: ________________

When to check breeding males: ________________

When to check house pets: ____________________

Other notes:

Deworming Schedules

When an animal is positive for:	Deworm again:	Recheck in:
Coccidia	_______ wks	_______ wks
Hookworms	_______ wks	_______ wks
Roundworms	_______ wks	_______ wks
Tapeworms	_______ wks	_______ wks
Whipworms	_______ wks	_______ wks

Tapeworms

Description: Two kinds of tapeworms infect both dogs and cats. One is transmitted by rodents, and the other is transmitted by fleas. The flea and the rodent are called the parasite's intermediate hosts. Control of the intermediate hosts is extremely important to prevent the reinfestation of tapeworms.

The adult tapeworm lives in the pet's intestine. It attaches to the intestinal wall and absorbs protein from the contents of the intestine. This is what we mean by a parasite living at the expense of another living being. Because the tapeworm is taking nutrition from the pet's intestine, the pet is not getting all the nourishment it needs.

Treatment: Adult tapeworms can be treated easily and effectively. The drugs come in both injectable form—for the doctor to give in the office—and tablet form—for the owner to give at home.

Prevention: Control of the intermediate host is a must. Fleas should be eradicated. Animals that regularly catch and eat rodents should be checked for tapeworms often.

Whipworms

Description: Whipworms usually occur only in dogs. Whipworms live in the large intestine and colon. They usually do not cause major illness unless the infection is severe. Clinical signs of whipworm infection include weight loss, poor haircoat, and a loose stool that may contain blood or mucus. Whipworms cannot be transmitted to humans.

Treatment: Whipworm eggs are detected by a fecal flotation test, although they can be more difficult to detect than hookworm and roundworm eggs. Whipworm infection is treated with one of several worm medications. Infested animals should be rechecked and/or dewormed again in several weeks.

Prevention: Once again, a clean yard free of stools and early detection are the best ways to prevent severe infestation. Daily and monthly oral medication is available and is often used in areas of frequent reinfection.

Heartworms

Description: The parasites we have discussed so far all live in the animal's intestines. As you might guess, heartworms live in an animal's heart and large blood vessels in the lungs. They primarily infect dogs, but occasionally a cat will be infected with heartworms.

The signs of heartworm infestation are similar to the signs of heart failure. These signs include tiring easily and a mild, nonproductive cough. In advanced cases of heartworm infestation these signs can be very severe.

Heartworms are transmitted from animal to animal by mosquitoes. For this reason, areas of the country with a lot of mosquitoes—such as warm climates and areas near water—experience worse problems with heartworms than areas with fewer mosquitoes.

Heartworms are detected by blood tests (see Chapter 10). X-rays of the chest can also be helpful to diagnose this parasite.

Life Cycle

1. Adult worms live in large blood vessels in the lungs and in the right side of the heart in infected animals.

2. Fertilized adult female worms produce microfilariae, which circulate in the blood.

3. A mosquito bites an infected dog, ingesting the microfilariae with the blood from the dog. (Infected cats generally don't have microfilariae.)

4. The mosquito bites and transmits mature larvae into a new host—an uninfected dog or cat.

5. The larvae migrate through the tissues to the

lung blood vessels and heart.

6. The larvae grow into adult worms in the lung blood vessels and heart.

Prevention: This is one case where an ounce of prevention is worth two pounds of cure.

Heartworm prevention in dogs and cats involves giving a daily or monthly medicine orally or topically at home. The medication should be continued throughout the mosquito season or throughout the entire year in areas severely infested with mosquitoes.

A dog must test negative for heartworms (with a blood test) before beginning preventive medication because an infected dog can have a serious, even fatal, reaction. Any dog taken off the medication during the cold winter months must test negative before beginning the medication again in the spring. Likewise, any dog over 6 months of age that is just starting the medication must first test negative for heartworm infestation. Cats can receive heartworm prevention without first being tested because they are less likely to have a reaction.

NOTE: Heartworm prevention is a prescription drug. Never sell it if you don't have a refill order on the patient's chart or if you're not absolutely certain that the dog has tested negative for heartworms within the last year.

Treatment: The two-part treatment for adult heartworms is serious and can be fatal to dogs. Treatment can be even more dangerous in cats, so the doctor usually will recommend supportive therapy instead.

The adult heartworm treatment consists of injections of a drug containing arsenic and hospitalization to monitor the pet. After a short stay in the hospital, the doctor will send the dog home and recommend rest. This is very important! This keeps the dog's blood pressure normal, which helps prevent

Clinic Policies on Heartworms

Prevention

How often to blood test dogs: ____________________

Types of Prevention

Monthly:	Dog's weight:	Medication amount:
______________	______________	______________
Daily:	**Dog's weight:**	**Size tab to take:**
______________	______________	______________

Treatment

Pretreatment tests needed: ______________________

____

Number of days of hospitalization: ______________

Microfilariae treatment:

Number of weeks after first treatment: ___________

Procedure during hospitalization: ______________

Final check or checks:

Number of days after microfilariae treatment: _____

Number of negative checks required: ____________

dead worms from forming a clot and blocking a major blood vessel in the lungs.

The treatment for microfilariae can be just as serious. The doctor will give the dog medicine and monitor it closely for shock caused by dying microfilariae. As soon as the dog is clear of microfilariae, the doctor will prescribe a prevention program. As previously mentioned, there are usually no microfilariae in the cat.

Horse Parasites

Intestinal parasites are a major cause of poor condition and poor health in horses. Even after a horse has been dewormed, reinfection is common because the life cycle of most horse parasites is direct—horse to pasture to horse. One horse with worms can easily infect an entire herd. In addition to the parasites described below, other equine parasites include large and small stomach worms, tapeworms, and threadworms.

The horse owner's goal should be to keep the parasite count as low as possible by switching the horse from pasture to pasture, feeding grain in feed buckets and hay in hay nets rather than feeding on the ground, and regular dewormings using alternating worm medicines. Deworming may be done with paste dewormers or by nasogastric or tube deworming. Unless otherwise indicated, these guidelines should be followed for the treatment and prevention of the parasites discussed below.

Bloodworms (*Large Strongyles*)

Large strongyles are the most dangerous group of equine intestinal parasites. As they migrate back to the intestines through the blood vessels, they often damage the blood vessel wall and cause an aneurysm. From this aneurysm, emboli or clots develop and inter-

Clinic Policies on Equine Parasite Control

Age to first deworm foals: ____________________

Recommended interval between routine dewormings:
For single (pet) horse: ____________________
For herd horses: ____________________
For show/performance horses: ____________________

Special requirements for breeding females:

Special requirements for pregnant females:

How often to do fecal checks:

rupt the main blood flow to the intestine. This causes the horse to develop colic. If the blood supply is cut off for a long time, the horse might die.

Bots (*Gasterophilus*)

This stomach parasite is common in most horses. Adult flies lay the yellowish eggs on the hairs of the horse's legs. Because the horse bites or licks its leg, attempting to remove the bothersome eggs, these larvae can irritate the tongue and gums. In addition, the adult parasites attach to the lining of the horse's stomach, creating shallow holes.

Pinworms (*Oxyuris*)

Pinworms are found in horses of all ages and irritate the mucosa of the colon as well as the area around the outside of the rectum. This causes the horse to scratch at the tailhead, often by rubbing against a fence or a tree. Other parasites that infect horses include large and small stomach worms, tapeworms, and threadworms.

Roundworms (*Ascarids*)

Roundworms are mostly found in colts and yearlings. They are large worms and can actually cause intestinal blockage in a young horse. During their life cycle, the larvae are coughed up from the lungs and reswallowed. Therefore, they can also complicate any existing respiratory condition.

Small Strongyles

Small strongyle parasites aren't as dangerous to the horse as the large strongyles. Their life cycle is similar, but they do not migrate beyond the intestines.

Treatment of Equine Intestinal Parasites

Treatment: A fecal flotation test diagnoses all of the

parasite eggs in the horse's stool. Worm medication may be given orally in a paste or liquid or administered by a nasogastric tube, directly into the stomach. Most horses are dewormed on a regular basis.

Prevention: A routine deworming program and pasture rotation allow the eggs and larvae to die out. A prescription food additive is available for daily use.

Cattle and Swine Parasites

Cattle and swine are usually raised commercially, as food animals. Every herd owner appreciates the value of routine parasite control, and effective, broad-spectrum deworming medicines are available for treatment and prevention of the parasites that commonly afflict cattle and swine. Routine deworming for all animals is highly recommended.

Clinic Policy on Cattle Deworming
Clinic Policy on Swine Deworming

CHAPTER

13

The Importance of External Parasite Control

Like the internal parasites discussed in the previous chapter, external parasites live at the expense of their hosts. The difference is that external parasites live on the *outside* of the body. Examples are fleas and ticks, which plague both dogs and cats. Ferrets, guinea pigs, and rabbits can become infested with fleas, especially if they have contact with an infested dog or cat. Ticks can also be a problem in horses' ears.

External Parasites

Fleas

Description: Fleas are small insects that take their meals from the blood of our pets. They are not limited to attacking pets, however. They bite humans as well. If you have ever been bitten by a flea, you know that it causes an uncomfortable reactive condition—it itches! Fleas can also transmit disease.

Fleas can make life miserable for a pet. Not only do they bite an animal, but they also run around on its dry, sensitive skin. Many animals are allergic to the flea saliva that is injected with each bite. This allergic reaction makes the itching worse.

Animals that become severely infested with fleas can develop flea anemia. This means that the fleas suck so much blood that the animal doesn't have enough to live on. Pale gums and weakness are the main signs of anemia. This is more common in puppies, cats, and smaller dogs because of their size, but it can also occur in large dogs.

Fleas can be hard to find. Many animals have thick fur, and fleas are small and run quickly when you are looking for them. However, they leave a telltale sign behind: flea dirt. These little black specks are actually flea excreta, or flea waste. Even though you may not be able to see a flea, flea dirt indicates that *fleas are present.*

Life Cycle

1. Adult flea.*
2. Adult flea lays eggs on the host.
3. Eggs fall off host and develop into larvae.*
4. Larvae become pupae with a cocoon. Nothing can kill the pupae at this stage.
5. Pupae develop into adult fleas.

* These stages are susceptible to insecticides.

The life cycle of the flea varies considerably in length, from 18 days to 20 months. *Warm temperatures and high humidity* speed up its life cycle. That is why fleas are more of a problem in southern than northern regions or desert areas.

Prevention and Treatment: The best defense is a good offense, and this is true of flea control. This is one area of veterinary medicine that has made giant progress moving into the new millennium. We can help our clients eliminate a pesky flea problem—but more important, we can prevent the problem from occurring in the first place.

We now have Insect Growth Regulators (IGR), sometimes referred to as Insect Development Inhibitors (IDI). There also are newer, safer insecticides that can be applied directly to the pet's skin. This vast array of new products include oral monthly tablets, topical monthly drops and sprays, immediate acting sprays, shampoos, collars, dips, and even an injection for cats that prevents fleas for up to six months. With this selection of products, environmental insecticides are rarely needed.

Every client coming through the door needs to know your veterinary clinic can offer a solution to prevent and control flea infestations. Familiarize yourself with each flea product available. A good idea for a staff meeting is for each employee to describe a product. How does it work? How long does it take to start working? Does it control or prevent other infestations? Can this product be used with other products?

Ticks

Description: A tick is a small insect that buries its head in an animal's skin, ingests a blood meal, and often transmits disease. This parasite attacks humans as well as pets. Rocky Mountain spotted fever and Lyme disease are transmitted to humans by ticks. In dogs, ticks transmit *Ehrlichia*, which can be fatal, as well as Rocky Mountain spotted fever and Lyme disease.

Like fleas, ticks can cause blood loss and anemia. It is not uncommon for animals to need a life-saving blood transfusion because of tick anemia.

There are several different kinds of ticks that range in size from small—smaller than a pinhead, to large—about the size of a pinky fingernail. All kinds are potentially harmful, and pets should be treated at the first sign of infestation.

Life Cycle:

1. Adult ticks attach to pets.
2. Ticks lay eggs.
3. In 30 days, the eggs hatch into larvae.*
4. The larvae develop into adult ticks.*

* These stages are treatable with insecticides.

The life cycle of the tick can range from two months to two years. High temperatures and humidity speed up its life cycle.

Treatment: To conquer and control tick infestations, the parasite must be eliminated on the host pet and in the environment. The important thing to remember about ticks is the 30-day incubation period of the eggs. The environment and the pet must be controlled for 30 days to break the tick's life cycle. Therefore, treatment must continue until the eggs have hatched and the insecticide can control the infestation.

Prevention: The new topical medications to prevent flea infestation can also prevent ticks. However, not every product is effective against ticks, so know your products. With these new choices, severe tick infestations can be prevented. The new medicines include topical monthly drops and sprays, new collars, and the traditional shampoos and dips.

Early treatment of pets will help prevent problems at the height of the tick season. Clients should examine their dogs for ticks regularly. Advise your clients to look inside their pet's ears, under their legs, and between their toes—all of the favorite hiding places for ticks. Pets should be treated before the first sign of ticks because the goal is to prevent this disease-carrying insect.

Notes

Clinic Flea and Tick Control Policies

For parasites on the pet

Flea-prevention pills or drops

For dogs: ______________________

For cats: ______________________

Topical products

For dogs: ______________________

For cats: ______________________

Months to treat (or year-round): ________________

Age to start treatment: ________________________

For parasites in the environment

Treatment for the house and/or yard: ___________

Recommended products for the yard: ___________

Recommended professional exterminator for heavy infestations: ___________________________________

CHAPTER

14

Dispensing Drugs and Supplies

A prescription drug is a chemical that is manufactured and sold to licensed professionals only. These drugs are used in the prevention and treatment of medical conditions. If used incorrectly, they can be harmful or even fatal.

A prescription for these drugs comes only from a doctor of medicine, or a doctor of veterinary medicine in our case. In order for this prescription to be valid, there must be an active doctor/patient relationship. This means the doctor examined the pet within the last year. However, many doctors feel more comfortable seeing their patients every six months.

What Can I Sell Without Asking the Doctor?

The products you sell in your job as veterinary receptionist fall into two categories: prescription and nonprescription. A prescription item is one that the doctor has designated as a course of treatment after examining the pet. A nonprescription item is a product the client may buy "over-the-counter," without having the pet examined by the doctor.

In general, you are free to sell any over-the-counter items. These include non-prescription dog and cat foods, pet vitamins, and most flea and tick remedies. Prescription items include heartworm tablets, specially prescribed oral medications, and prescription diets.

Refilling Prescriptions

When a client inquires about refilling a prescription, pull the client's chart to determine:

1. whether the prescription may be refilled without the doctor re-examining the pet

2. the exact name and correct strength of the medication that's been prescribed
3. how much of the medication to dispense
4. the correct dosage of medication

Be sure you know the doctor's method of coding refillable prescriptions on the patient chart so you won't keep the client waiting while you ask the doctor if a prescription may be refilled. Write the code to watch for in the space below.

OK to refill a prescription coded ______________

If the Prescription Has Been Approved for Refill

1. Go to the pharmacy area of your hospital, and locate the correct drug.
2. Double-check the name and strength of the medicine. Many drugs with the same name come in more than one strength, and many drugs have similar names.
3. Check the expiration date of the medicine. It will be printed somewhere on the label. Do not dispense drugs with expired dates; you should report any drugs nearing expiration to the doctor or the person in charge of ordering supplies for the clinic.
4. Count or measure the medicine carefully.
5. On the client's chart, note the date and the details of the prescription refill. For example: 6/31/00: refill Prednisone 20 mg. #30.
6. Prepare a prescription label. If your labels are computerized, you may only have to choose the correct drug and dosage, and the label will be printed out for you. WARNING: It's against the law to dispense prescription drugs without a proper label.
7. Package the drug in the appropriate container. Child-resistant packaging is recommended, and it is

required by law in some states.

8. If you prepare the label yourself, be sure to write it in terms the client will be able to understand. For example, if the doctor has written on the chart:

Tribrissen® (Mallinckrodt) 120 mg, 1 BID, #10

you must translate that to:

Give one tablet twice a day for five days. Tribrissen 120 mg. #10.

Be sure your instructions to the client are clear.

☛ TIP

It's a good idea to familiarize yourself with the pharmacy as soon as possible. How are the drugs arranged? Are they grouped according to type, with all the antibiotics on one shelf and all the topical ointments on another? Where are the eye drops and ear medications kept?

Then be sure you understand the doctor's prescription abbreviations. In the above example, the first word, Tribrissen, is the name of the drug. "120 mg" refers to the strength of the drug. Remember we said that many drugs with the same names come in different strengths—always double-check the strength of the prescribed drug. The next phrase on the prescription, "1 BID," refers to the dosage—in this case, one tablet twice a day. (A complete listing of prescription abbreviations appears at the end of this chapter.) The last part of the prescription, "#10," refers to the number of tablets you are to dispense.

NOTE: Your state board of veterinary medical examiners may have strict requirements about labeling prescriptions. Be sure you know what your state requires and follow the guidelines carefully. In many states, for example, a prescription label must display some or all of the following information.

1. the name, address, and telephone number of the clinic
2. the name of the veterinarian dispensing the medication
3. the names of the patient and client
4. the name of the medication or veterinary product
5. the quantity and strength of the product
6. directions for administration
7. the date dispensed
8. precautionary statements as required by law (for example, "not for human consumption," "poisonous," etc.)

Check your state requirements and post them in the pharmacy, along with a sample prescription label, so that all labels will be prepared correctly and consistently. Childproof lids should be put on all prescription containers unless the client specifically asks you not to do so.

Always remember to check a patient's chart before refilling a prescription. If the chart does not say the prescription may be refilled, check with the doctor before dispensing the medication.

If the Prescription Has *Not* Been Approved for Refill

When you pull the client's chart to see if the prescription may be refilled, you may see a note such as "Need to recheck Tuffy when medication runs out," "No refill until more lab work is done," or "OK to refill five times, then recheck." However it is phrased, this type of comment indicates that the doctor wants to see the pet before continuing a certain medication. There is a good reason for this: The doctor wants to evaluate the effect the medicine is having. After an evaluation, the doctor may choose to change the medication, change the dosage, discontinue it, or continue the original prescription. Your job, then, is to tell the client that the doctor would like to see the pet before refilling the prescription and then make an appointment for the pet.

For example, you might say, "So that we can make sure Fifi needs to continue with this medication, the doctor would like to recheck her. May I make an appointment for you?" If you are in doubt about refilling a prescription, *ask the doctor.* Never refill a prescription unless the chart specifically says you may do so.

☛ TIP

Give clients advance warning when a prescription is about to expire. For example, when refilling a prescription for the next-to-last time, tell the client, "After your next refill, the doctor will want to examine Buster to evaluate the effect of the medicine."

Heartworm Prevention

Most dogs are on medication to prevent heartworms, and we tend to take heartworm prevention for granted and treat it like a vitamin. But heartworm prevention is a prescribed medication, and a dog must be blood-tested negative for heartworms before the doctor can prescribe the medication for prevention. In some areas of the country where heartworms are a severe problem, doctors may require that dogs test negative every year in order to stay on the medication. You should not sell heartworm prevention to clients whose dogs have not been tested or whose most recent heartworm check cannot be verified at another clinic. Write your clinic's policy on selling heartworm prevention medication here:

Clinic Policy on Selling Heartworm Prevention Medication

Prescription Diets

Prescription diets are prescribed by the doctor to aid an animal's recovery from a specific medical problem. For example, an overweight dog may need to be on low-calorie food until it reaches its ideal weight. The doctor may then want to change foods. Or a cat with a urinary tract infection may need a special diet for a certain amount of time. The doctor may then want to recheck a urine sample to see if the diet is helping or if a change is required.

Always consult the patient chart before refilling prescription diets and note any refills on the chart. If in doubt, ask the doctor! Be sure you know the difference between prescription diets and everyday maintenance diets—which is which and where they are kept.

Prescription Flea and Tick Products

These newer and safer products are still prescriptions. As mentioned before, they require an active doctor/patient relationship. All the products are dosed by weight, so a recent and accurate weight of the pet is essential. Some products are affected by bathing the animal. Know your products!

Over-the-Counter Products

Leashes, collars, and nonprescription pet foods may be sold to anyone. If the purchaser is a regular client, you may want to note the purchase on the pet's chart. That way, when the owner comes in the next month and wants the same thing, you'll know what the product was. If you have a computer, record client product purchases there.

You can sell pet vitamins without a prescription,

as well as most external forms of flea and tick control, such as shampoos, sprays, and dips. But before you sell any flea products, take some time to learn about the products your clinic sells. Some products can be used safely on dogs but not on cats. Some products can be used together, while others cannot. Some—but not all—are safe for young animals. Some have a long residual effect—they will kill the fleas or ticks for a week or more after application—and some are strictly "immediate kill" products that offer only short-term effects.

Encourage your doctor to hold a staff meeting at which each staff member is responsible for describing one or two products. Hold these meetings two or three times a year because both staff members and products change.

☛ TIP

If you don't have a computer to keep track of client purchases, it is a good idea to note them on pets' charts. The next time they come in, you can ask how the product worked. It creates good will (you show that you care about their pets!) and will help you determine which of your products are getting the best results. Likewise, if the products you stock are not working, the doctor may want to use something else.

Prescription Abbreviations

SID	once a day
BID	twice a day
TID	three times a day
QID	four times a day
EOD	every other day
PRN	as needed
Q	every, as in Q 8 hr—every eight hours
Per os	by mouth
tab	tablet
cap	capsule
cc (liquid measure)	cubic centimeter (equals 1 ml)
ml (liquid measure)	milliliter (equals 1 cc)
HWP	heartworm prevention
RX	prescription
#	number of tablets to dispense

Notes

CHAPTER

15

Common Surgical Procedures

This chapter will familiarize you with the most common surgeries performed at a veterinary hospital. It is intended only to supplement your observations of these procedures to help you convey the value of surgery to your clients. Surgery looks easy when performed by a skilled surgeon, but it is a highly complex medical procedure, and its successful outcome depends on many factors.

The first of these is a healthy patient. Any pet about to have routine surgery should otherwise be in good health. A doctor predicts an animal's reaction to drugs, especially to anesthesia, based on knowledge of the reactions of other healthy animals. But an animal with bronchitis, for example, will have more difficulty breathing than a healthy animal and therefore is a surgical risk. Every animal that comes to your clinic for routine elective surgery will be thoroughly examined by the doctor to determine its ability to get through surgery without problems.

Another important factor that you must communicate to clients is that surgical patients must not eat before surgery. Many doctors advise clients to withhold food and water from a pet for at least 12 hours before surgery. Check your clinic's policy and notify clients of it. Always double-check when a client brings a pet in for surgery by asking if the pet ate or drank in the last 12 hours.

The reason for this strict requirement is that under anesthesia, a patient is totally relaxed. This includes the swallow reflex. An empty stomach helps prevent regurgitation, or vomiting, of stomach contents and the aspiration of the contents into the lungs. Stomach contents have a high acid level, and regurgitation and aspiration can cause death.

A third important item is the surgical consent form. No client should leave a patient for surgery at your clinic without having signed a consent form authorizing the doctor to perform the surgery. The form should state the client's name and address; the pet's name, species, and breed; and the surgical procedure to be performed. Always obtain a phone number where the client can be reached during the day in case the doctor has any questions. Fill in the chart at the end of this chapter to help you remember your clinic's policies surgical cases.

Where Is Surgery Performed?

Surgery is performed in sterile conditions in the surgery room. The word "sterile" as it pertains to surgery is important. When we talk about a sterile environment for surgery, we are talking about an absolutely clean and germ-free area. Being sterile is like being pregnant—either you are or you aren't! There is no in-between. This is why the surgery area is kept clean and disinfected and why traffic through the surgery area is prohibited.

Before surgery, both the doctor and the patient go through rigorous preparations. The doctor scrubs both hands and arms with antiseptic soap and then puts on a sterile surgical gown, cap, mask, and gloves. Once fully dressed for surgery, the doctor will not touch anything that hasn't been sterilized. Sterilization of instruments and surgical gowns is usually done in an autoclave. The autoclave has a pressurized chamber that uses high heat to kill bacteria and germs.

How Is Surgery Performed?

In the surgery room, the doctor carefully opens the sterile pack of surgical instruments. While the doctor is doing this, a veterinary assistant is preparing the animal for surgery. Usually this involves shaving the fur from the surgical site and scrubbing this area with antiseptic soap.

Some surgical procedures are performed with only a local or regional anesthetic. This means that the animal is awake but that the surgical site has been numbed. The doctor usually chooses this method for minor procedures or when the animal is an anesthetic risk. Some animals cannot withstand the effects of general anesthesia because of old age, respiratory problems, allergic reactions, and a variety of other reasons.

General anesthesia allows the animal to be asleep during surgery. Every veterinarian takes an oath to "temper pain with anesthesia," and most major surgery requires general anesthesia. In addition to preventing pain, general anesthesia keeps the patient from moving and relaxes muscle tension.

There are several different kinds of general anesthesia. These include injectables (either intramuscular or intravenous) and inhalation (gas). The gases are administered with oxygen through special anesthetic machines. For veterinary surgery, gas is the most commonly used form of anesthetic.

While under anesthesia, the patient is closely monitored with many devices. These monitors range from esophageal stethoscopes (a simple method to monitor heart rate and breathing) to sophisticated pulse oximeters, which monitor blood pressure, heart rate, and the level of oxygen in the blood.

Once the doctor has completed the surgical procedure, the animal's recovery is closely monitored. Many hospitals have a recovery area near the surgery room, while others use the kennel room for this purpose. In either case, the patient is watched to make sure that it wakes up without difficulty, that its breathing is normal, and that there is no excessive bleeding.

Pain management is another vastly improved area of veterinary medicine. As veterinarians educate their clients on the importance of pain management, many clients want to minimize their pets' pain with additional medicine. Some clinics allow authorization for extra pain medicine on their surgery consent form. Make sure you know the surgery policy.

Common Surgical Procedures

Ovariohysterectomy or Spay

The ovariohysterectomy (OHE), or spay, is the removal of the ovaries and uterus in the female. It is the same basic procedure for dogs and cats. OHE is usually called elective surgery because in most cases clients choose, or elect, to have their pets spayed. Occasionally a doctor will perform an emergency OHE to save the pet's life.

Spaying is a highly recommended operation because it reduces the risk of breast cancer and it prevents the female from going into heat and becoming pregnant. In a world overpopulated with dogs and cats, this procedure should be considered by every pet owner who is not in the dog- or cat-breeding business.

There are some misconceptions about the spay operation. It does not cause the animal to gain weight or change its personality. The procedure is equivalent to a complete hysterectomy for a woman and is considered major surgery.

NOTE: Check with your doctor about whether animals in heat may be spayed. Many veterinarians prefer to wait until the heat cycle has been completed. When the female animal goes into heat, the uterus enlarges to several times its normal size. The blood supply also enlarges to accommodate the extra tissue. An animal undergoing a spay operation while in heat has a higher risk for hemorrhaging, or bleeding uncontrollably.

☛ TIP

The care the animal receives when it goes home after surgery is critical to a good recovery. Print up home-care instructions for each procedure. Go over the instructions carefully with each client and always encourage the client to call if something—anything!—doesn't seem right.

Castration or Neuter

Castration, or neutering, is performed on males and is the removal of both testicles. In horses it is called gelding, which is why male neutered horses are called geldings. Castration in the male is recommended as strongly as the ovariohysterectomy is for females. It aids in pet population control, helps keep dogs from roaming because they do not follow the scent of every female in heat, and decreases a dog's incidence of prostrate problems.

Castration also diminishes or eliminates aggression, the male's tendency to "mark" a territory with urine, and obnoxious sexual behavior. This is particularly important in horses because stallions (unneutered male horses) can be difficult to handle—especially if there is a mare in heat nearby. Having a male animal neutered will not cause the animal to become fat and lazy.

Declawing Cats

As the name implies, declawing is the removal of the cat's claws and is recommended only for indoor cats. It can be performed on kittens or on adult cats. To prevent damage to their home furnishings, clients who plan to keep their cats strictly indoors should consider this surgery early in the cat's life. Most doctors recommend declawing the front feet only. Very little damage is done with the rear claws, and the cat still has some means of defense. Declawed cats can still climb small trees as long as they can get their paws partially around the tree trunk. This procedure is normally performed only on cats. Dogs are usually not declawed.

Ear Trim

An ear trim is a form of cosmetic surgery performed only on dogs. Some dogs, such as Doberman pinschers, are born with floppy ears, but the breed standard dictates that the ears should stand erect. Changing ears from hanging down to standing up can only be done surgically. This is elective cosmetic surgery and performed only on strong, healthy patients. Most doctors prefer to do ear trims on young dogs—usually those 9 to 12 weeks old. Older dogs' ears will thicken, which makes ear surgery much more difficult. Ask your doctor if this procedure is performed at your hospital.

Dewclaw Removal

The dewclaw in a dog or cat corresponds to the thumb in a human. It is located on the inside of the leg, higher than the other four toes, and does not bear any of the animal's weight. In dogs, dewclaws are often removed. They can cause problems for adult dogs if they catch in rugs or in debris outdoors. Often they tear and can become infected.

Dewclaw removal is considered minor surgery if it is performed when the puppy is young—*usually 3 to 5 days old.* At this age, the claws are very small, and the doctor can easily remove them. If it is done when the dog is older, it is treated as a major surgical procedure and the dog is given general anesthesia.

Tail Docking

Like ear trims, tail docking is breed-specific and strictly cosmetic. Certain dogs are born with long tails, but their breed standards dictate that the tails should be short. Tail docking is best done when puppies are 3 to 5 days old and is usually done at the same time as dewclaw removal. When it is done later in life, it becomes major surgery requiring general anesthesia and hospitalization.

Cesarean Section

A Cesarean or C-section is usually performed as emergency surgery when an animal is unable to give birth vaginally. It involves the surgical removal of puppies or kittens from the uterus.

Ovariohysterectomy for Pyometra

A pyometra is an infected uterus that is filled with pus. It is more common in dogs than in cats—especially in older, unspayed dogs—and is often first signaled by a vaginal discharge. The infection can be so extensive that a complete ovariohysterectomy (OHE) may be needed. However, the surgery is more difficult because it must be performed on a patient that is already in poor health from the uterine infection. The pet usually must stay in the hospital longer than would be required for a normal OHE. The risk of pyometra is another good reason for females to be spayed early in life.

Repair of Fractures

Fractures, or broken bones, may occasionally be set with a splint or a cast if the fracture is not too serious. However, many require surgical repair. With the animal under general anesthesia, the doctor may surgically pin the bone or affix a surgical plate to it in order for it to heal. This is called orthopedic surgery, and it can be complicated and demanding. Many doctors refer this type of surgery to orthopedic specialists. Ask your doctor about the policy at your clinic.

Tumor Removal

Just like people, animals suffer from cancer and tumors. They can be given chemotherapy, just like people, or the doctor may choose to remove it surgically. Small tumors are generally easier to remove than large ones. Any clients who ask about lumps they've found on their pets should be encouraged to come in for an examination as soon as possible.

Removal of Bladder Stones

Both dogs and cats can develop urinary bladder or urethral stones. The stones may irritate the lining of the bladder or uretha, causing painful, frequent urination with blood. Stones in the urethra can also cause a dangerous obstruction, resulting in an inability to urinate. Some bladder stones can be dissolved by a special diet. Other stones must be removed surgically. The stones are then analyzed to determine their cause and to make sure a proper program of prevention is maintained.

Clinic Surgical Policies

Procedure	Ideal age	In heat OK?	Withhold food for	# days in hosp.	Recheck due in	Suture rem. due	Vacc. req.	Lab req.
Spay								
Cat								
Dog								
Neuter								
Cat								
Dog								
Declaw								
Cats only								
Ear trim								
Doberman.								
Schnauzer								
Min. Pin.								
Bouvier								
Great Dane								
Boxer								
Pit Bull								
Dewclaws								
Tail Dock								

CHAPTER

16

Common Medical Problems

As we discussed in Chapter 4, much of your job will involve talking to pet owners who want you to diagnose their pets' medical problems. And to repeat the advice in Chapter 4, *never give medical advice to a client whose pet has not been examined by the doctor.*

However, you should have a basic knowledge of common medical problems and illnesses. It will help you to determine when something is an emergency and to better explain to clients why it is necessary for a doctor to see their pets. You can't talk confidently about something you're unfamiliar with, so here are some of the more common medical problems for dogs, cats, and horses.

Common Canine Problems

Anal Gland Impaction

The anal glands are located on each side of the rectum. They fill with fluid that is normally expressed or eliminated during a bowel movement. Anything that interferes with this normal draining process can cause the glands to become full, or "impacted," and will make the dog uncomfortable. Sometimes the impaction is bad enough to form an abscess. When a client tells you that his or her dog is "scooting," or dragging its rear end on the ground, it may be because the anal glands are impacted. To treat this problem, the doctor drains the glands, either manually or surgically. Sometimes the dog will need antibiotics. If the problem persists, the doctor may surgically remove the anal glands.

Bad Breath/Gingivitis/Tartar on Teeth

Just as your dentist cleans your teeth once or twice a year, dogs should have their teeth checked and cleaned regularly too. Dogs can suffer from tartar and plaque buildup on their teeth. This can lead to gingivitis (infection of the gums) and bad breath. When the gingivitis is advanced, the doctor will usually treat it with antibiotics and a teeth cleaning, using equipment much the same as what your dentist uses on you, to remove the plaque and tartar. Pets will receive anesthesia for safety.

Many clients have a hard time understanding why dogs—who don't eat sweets—need to have their teeth cleaned. However, years of eating soft canned food contributes to plaque and tartar buildup. Even pets who eat dry, crunchy food will accumulate the telltale yellow stains on their teeth.

Eventually this buildup leads to gingivitis. This gum infection bombards the animal's body with bacteria and poisons, and such infections have been linked to heart, kidney, and liver problems. In many cases, owners don't realize how bad their pets have been feeling until after they've had their teeth cleaned. Clients often report how much livelier and more playful their pets are once their teeth have been cleaned and the gum infection has subsided.

Clients should be encouraged to examine their pets' mouths regularly and should notify the doctor at the first signs of gum redness, bleeding gums, or buildup of yellow stains on the teeth. Better yet, encourage all clients to make regular cleaning part of their pets' routine care.

Check with your doctor on the protocols for thorough teeth cleanings. Because they require a general anesthesia, diagnostic tests may be indicated prior to the procedure.

Choking or "Asthma" Attack

When dogs have sinus congestion, they try to clear excess mucus by putting negative pressure at the back of their nasal passages. This is sometimes called "reverse sneezing." Dogs usually make a loud sound while they are inhaling to do this, a sound that frightens many owners into thinking that their dog is having a choking attack. Treatment is aimed at mucus reduction, usually with antihistamine, and with antibiotics if infection is present.

Ear Problems

Whenever a dog shakes its head constantly, scratches its ears, or holds one or both ears down, chances are good that it has an ear problem. Treatment depends on accurate diagnosis because what works on ear mites won't cure an ear infection!

Ear Mites: The doctor may find these by looking in the ear with an otoscope or by examining a swab of ear exudate (matter inside the ear) under a microscope. Ear mites are easily treated with special drops, but all pets in the same household must undergo the treatment at the same time to completely eliminate the problem.

Allergies: Ears are part of the skin, and many dogs experience repeated ear infections brought on by allergies. Routine cleansing of the ears, antibiotics, and steroids may all be included in the treatment.

Infection: Ear infections may develop because of ear mites, allergies, or other causes. Often the doctor will want to check for yeast or bacteria inside the ear to determine the exact cause of the problem. Antibiotics and cleansing solutions may be used in treatment.

Growths, Lumps, and Tumors

Owners who notice lumps on their pets should be encouraged to bring their pets in right away. Some lumps are cancerous, or malignant, and the doctor may want to remove these surgically before they get too large. In general, small lumps are easier to remove than large ones. The first step is for the doctor to examine the cells that make up the lump. This is done by extracting a few cells with a needle (a procedure called a needle aspirate) and examining them under a microscope. Some lumps—lipomas—are made of harmless fatty cells, but some are cancerous. Just as with humans, the sooner a tumor is removed, the better the chance for recovery.

Heart Failure

Heart failure is most common in older dogs. When the heart begins to fail, it doesn't pump as efficiently, and fluid often builds up in the lungs and in other body tissues. Major signs of heart failure include a nonproductive cough (nothing being coughed up) or a sudden swelling in the abdomen. The doctor uses ECGs, X-rays, and sonograms to diagnose this problem (see Chapter 10). Medication can reduce fluid buildup and help regulate the heart. Similar to the treatment in humans, a low-salt diet is often indicated.

Matting and Runny Eyes

Runny eyes have many causes, and the doctor should see the dog as soon as possible in order to make an accurate diagnosis. Causes of eye problems include allergies, disease, foreign bodies in the eye, ulcers in the eye, and malformed eyelids. Certain breeds, such as chows and Shar-Peis, may have inverted eyelids that cause the eyelashes to grow toward the eye, causing irritation. The treatment depends, of course, on the cause of the problem and includes antihistamines for allergies, antibiotics for infections, and surgery for malformation. The wrong medicine can often make the problem worse, so clients who want to buy ointment or drops for runny eyes must always see the doctor first.

Obesity

It's hard for people to resist giving their dogs treats and table scraps, but an overweight dog faces the same health risks as an overweight human. Excess weight puts a strain on the heart, can increase blood pressure, and may cause shortness of breath. The doctor measures body fat by feeling the dog's ribs. If the ribs can't be felt, the dog may be overweight. Many owners can help their pets lose weight by eliminating treats from their diet and cutting back on the amount of food they eat. But sometimes they need the help of a prescription reducing diet or other low-calorie food. When the doctor decides that a pet's weight is jeopardizing its health, he or she may prescribe one of these diets, rechecking the weight regularly until the pet reaches the desired weight.

Skin Problems

The skin is the largest organ of the body, and dogs seem to have a large number of skin problems. You will get many questions about itching, hair loss, red spots, and flaking. Once again, treatment depends on accurate diagnosis—there are as many treatments as there are problems! Here are a few of the more common skin problems:

Dry Skin: Major signs include dull hair and dry, flaky skin (dandruff). The dog often scratches a lot and can develop secondary bacterial infections. Treatment may include dietary supplements along with topical remedies, such as shampoos and conditioners. If a bacterial infection is present, antibiotic therapy may be needed.

Seborrhea: Major signs are patches of oily and dry skin and an unpleasant odor given off by the skin. A secondary bacterial or yeast skin infection sometimes develops. Treatment can include antibiotics, antifungals, dietary supplements, and shampoos.

Allergies: If a dog is allergic to something, the clinical signs often appear on the skin. Dogs can experience allergies to food, inhalants, and things in the environment. Treatment is aimed at controlling the clinical signs and includes antihistamines, shampoos, steroids, and dietary changes.

Demodectic (Red) Mange: This type of mange is usually found in adolescent dogs, and there may be an inherited predisposition to developing the disease. Clinical signs include patchy hair loss on the face and legs. The doctor diagnoses it with a skin scraping to detect the microscopic mites. Treatment, which is usually successful, can include dips or oral medications.

Sarcoptic Mange: People can catch this type of mange from dogs. Intense itching is the major sign of sarcoptic mange. It is diagnosed with a skin scraping, although it is often difficult to find. Treatment may include dips, injections, or oral or topical medications.

Ringworm: Ringworm is a skin disease caused by a fungus. The major sign is a circular, dry, scaly area of hair loss. There will be a ring of inflammation at the edge of the circular area. Ringworm is easily spread by direct contact and can be transmitted to humans. Therefore, treatment is aggressive and usually includes antifungal shampoos, topical medications, and oral medications.

Sore Throat/Tonsillitis

Dogs have tonsils, just as humans do. Signs of a sore throat or tonsillitis in a dog are frequent licking and swallowing and appetite loss. Treatment is usually aimed at the cause of the sore throat—an antihistamine if it is caused by an allergy and post-nasal drip, or antibiotics if it is caused by infection.

Feline Medical Problems

In addition to feline leukemia and FIP (discussed in Chapter 11), cats suffer from other common problems. Some of these include:

Abscesses

An abscess is an area of infection that is filled with pus. Often this area is swollen. Cats are prone to abscesses, and most result from cat fights. This is another reason to encourage clients to have their male cats neutered. Neutered cats are much less likely to fight than are intact cats. Clinical signs of abscesses include sudden swelling, usually in the head and neck area or around the tailhead, and a high temperature. Cats are often listless and refuse to eat. Treatment involves drainage of the abscess and a prescription of antibiotics.

Asthma

Cats suffer from allergies and may be susceptible to asthma. Clinical signs include a rapid respiratory rate and a "wheeze" the doctor hears while performing a chest exam. This problem can be fatal if not controlled. Treatment may include steroids and bronchodilators.

Feline Urinary Syndrome

Urinary problems occur in both male and female cats. An early warning sign is straining to urinate. The cat will make frequent trips to the litter box but will only pass a few drops of urine. The cat may urinate in inappropriate places, and owners may notice blood in the cat's urine. Male cats may have urethral obstruction which makes them unable to urinate. *This should always be treated as a medical emergency.* Treatment includes special diets and antibiotics. Blocked cats may have to be catheterized to allow them to urinate.

Growths, Lumps, and Tumors

Lumps on cats are often malignant. Unlike dogs, which suffer from a variety of benign lumps, including warts and lipomas, cats are more likely to have a serious problem if a lump is found. Lumps should be examined as soon as they are discovered (using a needle aspirate) or removed and sent to a lab for a complete examination, called a histopathology.

Heart Problems

If a cat has a rapid heart rate all the time, it may be suffering from heart problems. Sometimes the first sign of heart problems is a sudden weakness in the rear legs. The best way to make an accurate diagnosis is with a sonogram (see Chapter 10), and treatment varies depending on the diagnosis.

Hyperthyroidism

Cats can sometimes develop overactive thyroid glands. It is more common in older cats, and the main signs are weight loss and increased appetite. A blood test is necessary for diagnosis. Treatment may include pills, surgery, or radiation.

Megacolon or Massive Constipation

Signs of this problem include inability to have a bowel movement and an enlarged colon. Treatment consists of enemas designed to remove the obstruction (impacted fecal material) and often manual removal if enemas alone don't work. Cats suffering from constipation must be watched carefully to be sure that the problem does not recur. Often they must eat special diets and take stool softeners regularly.

Obesity

The "rib test" is done on cats as well as on dogs. If the doctor can't feel any ribs halfway down the rib cage, the cat may be overweight. In addition to heart strain and shortness of breath, cats can develop a problem called "fatty liver syndrome," which can be very dangerous. Weight loss should be gradual and is sometimes aided by prescription reducing diets and frequent weight checks.

Ringworm

The same fungus that causes ringworm in dogs also causes it in cats. But unlike dogs, who always show hair loss, cats with ringworm may not have any visible signs of infection—that is, they are asymptomatic ringworm carriers. This means the cat can carry the ringworm fungus, transmit it to humans and other animals, and never have any hair loss. This carrier state can be cured. Often when members of a family develop ringworm, the doctor will recommend that their cat be treated even if it is asymptomatic. Ringworm treatment for cats is aggressive, just as it is for dogs. Antifungal shampoos and topicals may be used, along with oral medication. Owners are often advised to clean contaminated areas of their houses with bleach or other antifungal cleansers.

NOTE: A client who has ringworm should be advised to call a family physician for the best course of treatment. Recommend that the pet be treated for ringworm, but never suggest methods of treatment for the client.

Equine Medical Problems

Colic

Colic refers to acute abdominal pain, which can have any number of causes. Introducing fresh grass into a horse's diet can cause colic, as can overeating and aneurysms caused by bloodworm migration. Colic should always be considered a serious problem until proved otherwise. Signs of colic include the horse turning and looking at its side, stretching out and standing in the stretched position, kicking at its stomach, or rolling or lying down. The method of treatment depends on the doctor's diagnosis of the type of colic. Colic is serious and should be considered a medical emergency.

Corneal Ulcer

This eye problem is signaled by pain in and around the eye; the horse will often keep the eye closed and will produce excessive tears. Early diagnosis is necessary to pinpoint the problem, and treatment depends on the diagnosis. Corneal ulcer is serious and should be considered a medical emergency.

Dentistry

If horses drop grain from their mouths while they are eating, they could be having problems with their teeth. Usually it means they are having pain while chewing, similar to what you feel if you bite your tongue or the inside of your cheek. The treatment is to "float" the teeth. This involves using a special file, called a dental float, to grind down the sharp points on the teeth. Horses need regular dental checks and their teeth should be floated whenever necessary. "Wasting" grain because of bad teeth can cause weight loss and poor health.

Founder (Laminitis)

Founder, or laminitis, is a result of the release of histamines to the blood vessels in the feet. When this occurs the blood vessels swell, which leads to pressure and pain. The first sign of founder may be lameness in both front feet. Treatment is aimed at reducing pain in the feet and shrinking the swollen blood vessels as early in the founder episode as possible. Founder is extremely serious and should be considered a medical emergency.

Limping

The major sign of limping is that the horse does not place 100 percent of its weight on the foot of the affected leg. When the lameness occurs in a front leg, a telltale sign is that the horse throws its head in the air when the sore foot is on the ground. The doctor performs a systematic exam beginning at the foot and going up the entire leg. Radiology can be extremely helpful in diagnosing lameness problems. Treatment depends on the cause of the problem and can range from hydrotherapy to the use of anti-inflammatory and painkilling drugs to surgery.

Obesity

The test for obesity in horses is the same as for

dogs and cats. The doctor should be able to feel the horse's ribs. A horse that cannot lose weight no matter how conscientious the owner is about diet may have a thyroid problem and should be checked; this requires a blood test.

Notes

CHAPTER

17

Commonly Asked Questions: Small Animals

This chapter contains some of the questions (grouped according to subject matter) that veterinary receptionists are commonly asked. Study this handbook thoroughly, and you'll already be able to answer most of them! Each question has been answered appropriately in a short and simple style. Remember, this is you, the receptionist, talking—not the doctor.

In many instances, blanks have been left so that you can customize the answer to fit your clinic's specific policies. Space has been left at the end of each section for you to jot down questions frequently asked at your clinic (if they are not included here), along with the best response. Experienced receptionists may find this especially helpful in training new staff members.

Remember that when a client asks you questions about your services, your main goal—in addition to educating the owner—is to make an appointment for the pet. The natural last line to many of the answers here is, "May I make an appointment for you so we can take care of that?"

Keep in mind that many questions will be about prices, so keep your price information handy. Because price information is specific to each clinic, such questions are not included here.

Immunization Questions

Q: How old does my pet have to be for a rabies shot?

A: The doctor normally gives the rabies shot at __________ months of age. We also recommend vaccinating against canine distemper and parvovirus (feline distemper and feline leukemia).

Q: How old should my puppy (or kitten) be to start its shots?

A: We recommend starting the vaccinations

at ________ weeks of age. We give them in a series _____weeks apart so that your pet will have good immunity.

Q: Why is a series of shots necessary? Will my pet have to have the series every year?
A: The series of vaccinations helps ensure a high level of protective immunity in a young pet. This is the age when they are most susceptible to many contagious diseases. Once they are grown they will need yearly boosters of their vaccinations but will not need to repeat the series.

Q: Can my puppy catch distemper (parvovirus) even though it has started its shots?
A: A puppy's immunity is not complete until it has finished the entire series of puppy vaccinations. Until your puppy has developed a more complete immunity through its series of vaccinations, it is at risk and may possibly become infected.

Q: Why does my dog need shots other than the rabies shot?
A: There are several highly contagious dog diseases that we can protect your dog from through vaccination. Because most of these diseases are fatal, we want to give your pet the best protection.

Q: What is canine distemper?
A: Distemper is a highly contagious disease among dogs. It is almost always fatal. Although it is more common in puppies than in adult dogs, all dogs are susceptible to it. We recommend vaccinating your dog yearly because canine distemper is an extremely dangerous disease.

Q: What is parvovirus?
A: Parvovirus is a highly contagious viral disease among dogs. It causes vomiting and bloody diarrhea.

Because we now have a vaccine against this deadly disease, we recommend protecting your dog yearly when it has its annual vaccinations.

Q: How can you tell if an animal has rabies?
A: The clinical signs of rabies vary, and the old stories about animals foaming at the mouth are not always true. If you suspect that your pet has been exposed to rabies or has been bitten by a rabid animal, you should bring it to the doctor immediately for examination—for your pet's protection as well as your own.

Q: Why can't I vaccinate my own pet for rabies?
A: State law requires that a licensed veterinarian give the rabies vaccination to be sure it has been administered properly and for accurate record-keeping purposes. Rabies is still a serious problem, and rabies-control officers keep accurate records of the number of rabies vaccinations given and the type of vaccine used. If your pet ever bites someone, the doctor will be able to attest to the fact that the vaccine was administered properly and that the pet is inoculated against rabies.

Q: How often does my pet need to be vaccinated?
A: Most veterinarians recommend yearly vaccinations to maintain a proper level of protective immunity in pets, but check with your doctor to be sure. And some rabies vaccines are licensed for use every three years.

NOTE: There is no single correct answer to this question. The frequency of vaccination depends on the disease agent involved, the age and health of the pet, and the pet's risk of contracting the disease.

Q: My dog was exposed to distemper (parvovirus). Will he catch it? How can I be sure he doesn't?

A: If your dog has been vaccinated against distemper (parvovirus), he should be protected, but we recommend a booster vaccination in cases of direct exposure. If your pet has never been vaccinated, you should bring him in immediately for shots since these offer the best chance of resisting the disease.

Q: Can I catch Lyme disease from my dog?
A: Studies show that the disease is not directly transmitted from dogs to humans. Lyme disease is transmitted by ticks. If your dog has ticks, you may run a risk of being bitten by one, too. You can catch Lyme disease from a tick only, not from your dog.

Q: Can I catch feline leukemia from my cat?
A: To date there have been no documented cases of feline leukemia being transmitted to people, nor any higher incidence of leukemia in people with cats. However, if your cat tests positive for feline leukemia, we recommend that you talk with the veterinarian.

Q: Can I get my cat vaccinated for feline leukemia without having it tested first?
A: Write in your clinic policy here:

Clinic Policy on Feline Leukemia Vaccinations

Q: My cat stays inside all the time. Why does it need vaccinations?
A: If you ever have a personal emergency requiring you to board your cat or a medical emergency

requiring you to hospitalize your cat, the unvaccinated cat will be vulnerable to any of the feline diseases. It may be even more susceptible than other cats because it has never been exposed to any type of disease.

Q: Is FIV in cats the same as HIV in humans? Could I possibly catch AIDS from my cat?

A: FIV affects the cat's immune system, but to date there have been no documented cases of FIV being transmitted to people, nor of people contracting AIDS from cats.

Q: We have adopted a stray cat. Should I do anything special before I let it play with my other cats?

A: You should have the new cat examined by the veterinarian before exposing it to your other cats. The new cat should be tested for FIV and feline leukemia—two deadly diseases that could be transmitted to your cats. Also, we strongly recommend that you have your new cat vaccinated as soon as possible. (See Chapter 11.)

Other Immunization Questions

Internal Parasite Questions

Q: What is a parasite?
A: A parasite is an organism that lives at the expense of another living being. In our pets, these usually take the form of intestinal worms (internal parasites) and fleas and ticks (external parasites).

Q: How can I tell if my pet has worms?
A: Some parasites, such as tapeworms, are visible to the naked eye, but others must be detected under the microscope. If you will bring in a stool specimen, we will be glad to examine it microscopically to see if your pet has worms.

Q: What are heartworms, and how do I tell if my pet has them?
A: Heartworms are parasites that live in the animal's heart or in large blood vessels in the lungs. To test for heartworms, we draw a small blood sample and examine it under the microscope or run a special test (see Chapter 10). (Ask your doctor about your clinic's protocol.) Heartworms can be prevented easily using medication, but we have to be sure your pet tests negative before beginning the prevention.

Q: What causes heartworms?
A: Heartworms are transmitted by mosquitoes. If a mosquito bites a dog that is infected with heartworms and then bites your dog or cat, your pet could become infected with heartworms. We highly recommend that all dogs take medication for heartworm prevention to keep this from happening. Heartworm preventive medications are also available for cats.

Q: How often should my dog be tested?
A: In our area, we recommend that your dog be checked for heartworms __________ times a year.

Q: I forgot to give my dog its monthly heartworm pill last month. What should I do?

A: We recommend (choose your clinic's recommendation): that you *give/do not give* this month's pill as usual. In _______ months we will want to test your dog for heartworms to be sure it's still negative.

Q: I forgot to give my dog its daily heartworm prevention. What should I do?

A: Write your clinic's policy here:

Clinic Heartworm Prevention Policy

Q: Can I get worms from my pet?

A: Under normal sanitary conditions, no. But if people play or work in areas contaminated with feces, they can run the risk of contracting internal parasites. Children are more susceptible because they often play with dirt or in sandboxes and then put their hands into their mouths.

Q: Can I catch anything by cleaning out my cat's litter box?

A: *Toxoplasma* oocysts pass out in the feces of cats and can cause problems if transmitted to pregnant women. That's why pregnant women and immunosuppressed individuals should not clean out litter boxes. With normal sanitary precautions, litter boxes pose no problem for other people.

Q: Where do adult pets get worms?
A: Most intestinal parasites are transmitted in the pet's stool. When a dog steps in contaminated stool or ingests the egg, the parasite enters his body. Keeping the yard clean and having your pet checked for worms regularly will prevent most parasite infestation. Heartworms are transmitted by mosquitoes. Testing your dog for heartworm infection and keeping him on heartworm prevention will prevent heartworms from becoming a problem.

Q: How often should I deworm my pet?
A: We recommend a stool check ________ times a year to see if your pet has a parasite problem. There is no need to deworm unless your pet actually has worms.

Q: My dog has been scooting its behind on the floor. Does that mean it has worms?
A: Scooting can be a sign of tapeworms. We recommend that you examine your pet closely for signs of tapeworm infection. Tapeworm segments pass out of the pet's rectum and often catch in the fur on the legs and tail. If tapeworms are not the problem, the doctor will look for another cause, such as impacted or infected anal glands.

Q: My dog has diarrhea. Does that mean he has worms?
A: Worms often cause diarrhea, and we recommend a stool check and a physical exam to

determine what the problem is. Diarrhea can debilitate a dog quickly and should be controlled as soon as possible.

Q: What are these little white segments I've been noticing in the fur on my pet's legs and tail?

A: You are most likely seeing tapeworm segments that are becoming stuck in the hair when they pass out in a bowel movement. We recommend that you bring us a sample segment, if possible, so we can determine which kind of tapeworm your pet has. We can then deworm your pet and help you prevent it from getting them again.

Other Internal Parasite Questions

External Parasite Questions

Before you answer any flea and tick questions, make it your job to do two things:

1. Educate your clients about your flea and tick products. Many people still do not know that their veterinarian carries a complete line of flea- and tick-control products.
2. Be sure you understand that effective flea and

tick control depends on eliminating the parasites from the pet *and* the environment. If either step is missing, the control program will be ineffective.

Q: How can I get rid of my pet's fleas (or ticks)?
A: It's very hard to eliminate fleas and ticks altogether, but I can help you with an effective control program. The key to success is to treat your pet and the environment at the same time. There are monthly pills that will help keep fleas from reproducing on your pet. We also recommend that you bathe and dip your pet, fog or spray your house, and spray your yard—all on the same day. You will have to do this at regular intervals to break the life cycle of the fleas and ticks. Why don't you come by and let me show you our flea- and tick-control products, and we can devise a control program suited to your needs.

Q: I sprayed my yard and house, and I bathed my dog like you said three weeks ago, but the fleas are back, worse than ever! What went wrong, and what else can I do?
A: One treatment rarely gets rid of a flea or tick problem. Continued treatment at regular intervals, usually weekly at first, is needed to get the problem under control. Fleas (and ticks) in their immature stages are very hard to kill, and their continual hatching is why you may still be seeing them.

Q: I don't like the smell of insecticides in the house and I don't think it's safe for children. What else can I do?
A: Many exterminating companies now offer borax treatment. This is a noninsecticidal powder that's applied to your carpets just once a year and keeps fleas from reproducing in your house.

Q: Can I use my dog dip on my cat?

A: Always read the label carefully before using any product on your dog or cat. Many dog dips are too strong for cats. If the label says, "Not for use on cats," don't use it! If you are still in doubt, bring it in and let us double-check it for you. There are some alternatives to dip, such as flea combs, shampoos, sprays, and powders.

Q: How often can I dip my pet?
A: Check the label on the dip. It should tell you exactly how often you can use it. If you have any doubts, bring it in and let us look at it.

Q: How old should my pet be before I dip it?
A: Dips contain strong insecticides, and great care must be taken in using them on young animals. In general, no animal under 6 weeks of age should be dipped. Read the label carefully to see if your dip is safe to use on a young pet. If you don't already have dip at home, let us recommend a safe one for you.

Q: If I can't dip a young pet, how can I treat newborns for fleas?
A: There are several products that are safe for use on newborn puppies and kittens as long as they are used correctly. I'll be glad to show you how to treat your young puppies or kittens with some of the products we have here.

Q: How long do I have to keep my dog out of the yard after I spray the yard with insecticide?
A: The label on the insecticide bottle should tell you the safe amount of time to keep your pet out of the yard. If it doesn't, a good rule to follow is to wait until the insecticide has totally dried before letting your pet out. If you apply granules, water them thoroughly, and let the yard dry before you let your pet go outside.

Q: How can I tell if my dog has the kind of ticks that will give me Rocky Mountain spotted fever or Lyme disease?

A: It's hard to tell the difference between ticks. Unless we send the tick to the state laboratory for testing, there isn't really any way to tell. We certainly recommend testing a tick that bites you or a family member. Otherwise, it is best to keep your dog as free of ticks as possible through bathing and dipping and treating the environment.

Q: My pet scratches constantly. Does it have fleas?

A: Constant scratching can be a sign of flea infestation, but it might also mean your pet has dry skin or possibly even a medical problem, such as an allergy. If the scratching continues in spite of careful flea control, we recommend a visit to the doctor to determine the cause of the itching.

Q: Can I catch ringworm from my cat? And how should I cure my cat of ringworm?

A: Ringworm is not really a worm at all—it's a fungus. And, yes, it is contagious to humans. At the first sign of ringworm in your cat, bring it in so the doctor can prescribe medicine, shampoo, or ointment. Call your family doctor to ask how to prevent or cure the problem in yourself.

NOTE: This is important to remember. Whenever clients present you with human ailments—whether it's ringworm, a dog bite, or a cat scratch—refer them to their family doctor. Never prescribe treatments for clients! Some problems may be more serious than they sound on the phone, and advice from you could prevent someone from seeking proper treatment.

Reproduction Questions

Questions About Females

Q: Won't my pet get fat and lazy if I spay her?

A: The spaying operation *does not* contribute to obesity in dogs or cats at all. If you watch her diet and give her plenty of opportunity for exercise, you shouldn't have a problem.

Q: At what age can I have my pet spayed?

A: The doctor recommends spaying your female at ______ months of age. It's best if she (choose one): *does/does not/doesn't matter* complete one heat cycle first. Before we can do the surgery, she must be current on her vaccinations and test negative for worms and heartworms.

Q: Will my female still come in heat after spaying?

A: No. The spaying operation will eliminate heat cycles.

Q: Will she be able to get pregnant after spaying?

A: No. The spaying operation removes the ovaries and the uterus. Therefore she will be infertile and won't be able to get pregnant.

Q: Can my female pet be spayed while she is in heat or while she's pregnant?

A: This must be answered according to your clinic's policy. If the answer is yes, you might say, "We can do the surgery while she is in heat or pregnant, but it takes a little longer, and we charge a little bit more for it. If she is far into her pregnancy, it would be best to let the doctor examine her to determine whether the surgery should be done and how much it will cost." If the answer is no, you might say, "The doctor prefers that you wait until she is out of heat (until the puppies or kittens are born)."

Q: How soon after my dog/cat has puppies/kittens do you recommend that she be spayed?
A: As soon as the puppies or kittens are weaned and the mother's milk has dried up, she can be spayed.

Q: How can I help to dry up my pet's milk now that her puppies (or kittens) are weaned?
A: Reducing the amount that she eats and drinks will help to dry up her milk. Be sure that she is separated from the puppies (or kittens), and feed her smaller amounts of food than normal for several days.

Q: Why should I have my pet spayed?
A: Spaying is the best form of pet population control. In addition, it eliminates messy heat cycles and prevents unwanted litters. Other important reasons to spay your pet are that spaying lowers the chance of breast cancer later in life and eliminates the chance of pyometra, a life-threatening uterine infection.

Q: How often does a female dog come in heat?
A: Female dogs usually come in heat twice a year.

Q: How long does a female dog stay in heat?
A: The heat cycle usually takes about three weeks to complete.

Q: How often does a female cat come in heat?
A: Cats come into heat seasonally. They cycle at approximately 21-day intervals during the spring, summer, and fall.

Q: At what stage in the heat cycle should I breed my female cat?

A: Cats are spontaneous ovulators. This means they ovulate spontaneously after being bred. Therefore, the timing of mating during the heat cycle isn't critical in cats.

Q: Does my female have to have a litter to be a better pet?
A: No. In fact, more heat cycles and pregnancies increase the chances of mammary tumors later in life.

Q: When can I first breed my female dog?
A: For a planned breeding, we recommend you wait until the second or third heat cycle.

Q: At what stage in the heat cycle should I breed my female dog?
A: The fertile portion of the heat cycle is usually during the second week of heat or about the ninth day from the beginning of heat. The fertile period normally lasts several days and is characterized by the female "standing" for the male. The doctor can make scrapings of the vaginal wall to determine the time of ovulation.

Q: How long does a female dog stay pregnant?
A: The gestation period for a female dog is about 62 to 63 days.

Q: How long does a female cat stay pregnant?
A: The gestation period for a cat can be from 59 to 68 days and is usually about 63 days.

Q: I'm not sure when my dog was bred. Is there a way to tell when she will have the puppies?
A: Yes, the doctor can examine her to make sure it is not a false pregnancy, which is a common problem, and predict about when she is due. He will also explain the whelping (delivery) procedure.

Q: I'm not sure when my female cat was bred. How can I tell when the kittens will be born?

A: We recommend a prenatal checkup for the doctor to estimate the delivery date and the number of kittens, as well as to recommend vitamins or other special care. Unlike dogs, cats do not have false pregnancies.

Q: How soon does a cat come back in heat after she's had a litter of kittens?

A: Cats can sometimes come back into heat while nursing a litter, so it's important to keep them away from male cats until they can be spayed.

Q: If my registered female dog is bred by a stray dog, will this affect her future litters?

A: No, each litter is separate and there is no carryover between litters. However, care should always be taken to prevent unwanted puppies.

Q: How can I tell when my female dog is ready to deliver puppies?

A: Delivery in a female dog is called whelping. The first stage of labor is the dropping of body temperature. Let me arrange a visit for you so the doctor can explain what to expect and how to tell if there is trouble.

Q: How long will it take my dog (or cat) to give birth to her litter?

A: The length of time varies from animal to animal, but if your pet is in hard labor for an hour with no sign of a puppy (or kitten) being born, she may be having a problem. Call the doctor if this happens.

Q: Is it possible for a litter to have different fathers?

A: Yes, if there are five offspring, it is possible there could be five different fathers.

Q: My female dog has just been bred, and I don't want a litter. What should I do?

A: Bring her to the office as soon as possible. The doctor will examine her to see if there is actually a chance for puppies. This is done with a vaginal scraping to detect the presence of sperm and to determine the time of ovulation. There are several alternatives to terminating unwanted pregnancy, which the doctor will discuss with you.

Q: What is a false pregnancy?

A: False pregnancies occur in dogs, usually after a normal heat cycle. The dog's hormones trick her into thinking she is pregnant when actually she is not. A female with a false pregnancy will often make a nest in which to have puppies, carry stuffed animals in her mouth, and even produce milk. False pregnancy can be treated during an office visit, and the doctor will explain more about it at that time.

Questions About Males

Q: At what age should I have my pet neutered?

A: The doctor recommends neutering at about _____ months of age.

Q: Why should I have my pet neutered? Do you recommend neutering?

A: Yes, we do recommend it. Neutering the male helps control pet overpopulation. Neutering also helps prevent your pet from fighting with other males, decreases his aggressiveness, may help decrease his territorial marking behavior, helps keep him at home, stops unwanted sexual activity, and decreases the incidence of health problems related to the reproductive organs.

Q: Will neutering make my pet fat and lazy?

A: No. What it will do is prevent your pet from

roaming the neighborhood in search of a female in heat. If you watch his diet and give him plenty of chances for exercise, he should experience only natural weight gain.

Q: My dog has become aggressive and rough. Will neutering help stop that?
A: Neutering has been shown to decrease aggressiveness in dogs and make them better pets.

Q: If I neuter my cat, will he stop spraying my furniture?
A: When a cat sprays, he is exhibiting the male tendency to mark his territory with urine. Neutering decreases his male hormones and makes him much less likely to exhibit this undesirable trait.

Q: Couldn't I just give my dog a vasectomy? Why does he have to be castrated?
A: A vasectomy makes your dog incapable of breeding, but does nothing to diminish his sexual drive. He will still roam, fight with other dogs, and tend to be aggressive. By castrating, you reduce the hormones that are causing the undesirable behaviors. You also eliminate his chance for developing testicular cancer.

Q: How old does my dog have to be to be used for stud?
A: Dogs vary in the length of time it takes them to reach sexual maturity. Generally a dog that is 1 1/2 to 2 years old is ready to be used for stud.

Q: Why do dogs "tie" or stick together when breeding?
A: This occurs because of an enlargement in the male. It acts as a plug to keep the sperm from falling out and increase the chances of conception.

Q: How can I separate breeding dogs that are stuck together?

A: Please be patient and calm. The breeding "tie" is a natural phenomenon, and anything you do to scare the dogs could hurt them. With time they will separate.

Other Reproduction Questions

Medical Questions

It is important to remember that when a client describes a sign to you and asks you what the problem is, you must always say, "The doctor will need to see your pet to determine exactly what the problem is." The answer to each question below dealing with clinical signs should always begin or end with that statement.

Q: How do you take an animal's temperature?

A: Use a standard or digital lubricated rectal thermometer for about three minutes (or until the digital thermometer signals the reading is complete).

Q: What is a dog's normal temperature?
A: A dog's normal temperature sometimes varies but is usually about 101.5 degrees Fahrenheit.

Q: What is a cat's normal temperature?
A: A cat's normal temperature sometimes varies but is usually about 101.5 degrees Fahrenheit.

Q: My pet's teeth are falling out. Is that normal?
A: Puppies and kittens have "baby teeth" just like humans. It is normal for them to lose these first teeth when they are about 3 1/2 months old to make room for their adult teeth. Look inside your pet's mouth and be sure a baby tooth has fallen out wherever you see a new tooth coming in. If the baby teeth don't fall out, they may have to be pulled.

Q: I can't get my pet to eat, no matter what I feed him. Is there anything I can do?
A: If your pet is playful and acting normal in every other way, it is probably nothing to worry about. If it seems listless and droopy, it should be checked by the doctor. If you are offering your pet a balanced food and plenty of fresh water every day, it is highly unlikely he will starve himself to death. When he is hungry, he will eat.

Q: My pet seems to spend an awful lot of time sleeping. Is that normal?
A: Yes. Puppies and kittens both require lots of rest, just like human babies do. However, they should have periods of activity in between the times they are resting. If you feel that your pet may be too inactive, we should give it a thorough checkup and make sure it doesn't have worms.

Q: My dog has been out in the hot weather all day,

and now he seems to be panting quite hard. What should I do?

A: Dogs cool off by panting; it exchanges warm air for cool air and evaporates water from the mouth, tongue, and lungs. You may help him cool down by putting ice cubes in his water bowl or by wetting him with cool water. If your dog also exhibits weakness, and a rectal temperature above 104 degrees Fahrenheit, he may have heat stroke. Put cool, wet towels around him and bring him into the clinic immediately.

Q: It's going to be extremely cold tonight, and my dog stays outside. Is there anything special I should do for him?

A: Dogs need protection from extremely cold nights. Shorthaired dogs need more protection than double-coated or longhaired dogs. Light bulbs can be hung in the dog house for heat, or you may want to bring your dog into the garage, basement, or laundry room for the night.

Q: Why is my dog scooting its rear end on the floor?

A: Scooting can be a sign of anal-gland problems, or it may mean that your dog has tapeworms.

Q: My dog has been coughing for several days. What should I do?

A: A cough can be caused by a number of things, such as allergies, bronchitis, or even kennel cough. The doctor should check your dog so we can determine the cause of the problem.

Q: My dog is breathing heavily and seems uncomfortable. What could the problem be?

A: Labored breathing can be a sign of heartworms, respiratory problems, or heart failure. The doctor needs to look at your dog as soon as possible.

Q: Why does my dog have such bad breath?
A: Bad breath can be a sign of gum infection and teeth problems.

Q: My pet is having trouble chewing. What is the problem?
A: If your pet's teeth need cleaning and if the gums are infected, it might be painful for him to chew. Ulcers or infections in the mouth can also cause this.

Q: My pet has runny eyes, but I don't see anything in the eye. Do I need to bring him in?
A: Yes. Runny eyes can be caused by allergies, illness, injury, and infection. The doctor must examine your pet to determine the cause.

Q: My pet seems to be getting fat. Should I be worried?
A: Weight gain can be harmful if left unchecked. Let's make an appointment for a weight check so you can discuss your pet's diet with the doctor.

Q: My dog seems to be losing its hair. Is there a special kind of dip I should buy?
A: A dip may be what you need, but we won't know until the doctor finds out why your dog is losing its hair. Some hair loss is due to allergies, illness, or other causes.

Q: My pet scratches at herself constantly. I don't see any fleas on her. What is the problem?
A: Sometimes itching is caused by allergies or mange. Once the doctor determines the cause of the itching, we can treat it.

Q: Why does my dog chew at its feet?
A: This is almost always a sign of an allergy.

Q: Why has my dog chewed a big bare patch near its tail?
A: It's probably itching due to fleas or an allergy.

Q: All of a sudden, my dog can't jump on the couch or go up and down the stairs. What's wrong?
A: That can be a sign of a back problem, and this is often quite painful for your pet.

Q: My cat is limping. He sleeps all the time and won't eat.
A: He might have an abscess and may need antibiotics.

Q: My dog keeps shaking its head and scratching its ears. Can I come in and pick up some ear drops?
A: The doctor can't determine what medicine you'll need until the cause of the ear problem is known.

Emergency Questions

Q: My pet has licked up some antifreeze. Will this hurt him?
A: Antifreeze is extremely poisonous to dogs and cats. Please bring him to the clinic immediately for treatment.

Q: My pet has gotten into rat poison. Will it hurt him?
A: Rat poison can cause serious blood-clotting problems in dogs and cats. He should be brought in as soon as possible.

Q: My cat stepped in turpentine and then licked it off his paws. Now he seems to be foaming at the mouth. What should I do?
A: Turpentine and other tar products are toxic to cats. Please bring him in immediately for treatment.

Q: My pet was just hit by a car. What should I do?
A: Make sure it has an open airway and can breathe. If your pet is a dog, secure its mouth to prevent biting—a stocking works well as a temporary muzzle—and transport it to the clinic on a board to control its movements and prevent further injury. If it is a cat, put it in a box. Bring the pet to the clinic as soon as you can, even if you think it is fine. Sometimes an injury can cause internal problems that aren't readily apparent.

Q: My cat is chewing on my cane plant. Will it hurt him?
A: Yes. In fact, most ornamental plants are toxic to cats.

Q: My pet has had diarrhea for a couple of days. What's causing it, and what should I do?
A: Diarrhea can be caused by illness, worms, digestive upset, or poison. If your pet has diarrhea, there is always danger of dehydration. Bring in your pet as soon as possible for treatment.

Q: My pet has been vomiting. What should I do?
A: Vomiting can be caused by illness, digestive upset, or poison. With vomiting, there is always danger of dehydration. Bring in your pet for treatment as soon as possible.

Q: My dog's abdomen suddenly became extremely bloated, and now he looks very uncomfortable. What should I do?
A: There is a condition in dogs called bloat. This is where the stomach becomes filled with gas. Bloat is considered a medical emergency and should be treated immediately.

Q: My cat goes to the litter box constantly, but little or no urine comes out. What should I do?

A: Your cat may have a urinary tract infection or may have a blockage that's preventing it from urinating. You should bring him to the clinic immediately.

Other Emergency Questions

CHAPTER

18

Commonly Asked Questions: Horses

Immunization Questions

Q: How old does my newborn foal have to be to start vaccinations?
A: A tetanus antitoxin should be given immediately after birth, and the other immunizations should be given when the horse is ______ weeks of age.

Q: Why does a horse need a rabies shot?
A: Horses are exposed to wild animals that carry rabies, just as dogs and cats are. Horses that spend any amount of time in a pasture should be protected against rabies.

Q: How can you tell if a horse has rabies?
A: The first sign may be an abnormal gait. Signs progress over several days. If there is any reason to suspect the horse has been exposed to rabies, the doctor should examine it immediately.

Q: Is a series of vaccinations necessary for a young horse?
A: To provide full immunity, a young horse needs the initial vaccination series. After that, the horse will need annual boosters to maintain immunity.

Q: My horse is never around other horses. Why does it need to be vaccinated?
A: Not all diseases are transmitted by direct contact with horses. Tetanus is caused by bacteria entering a puncture wound, and sleeping sickness is transmitted by mosquitoes.

Q: Can I catch flu from my horse?
A: Although the clinical signs of equine flu are similar to human flu, there is no evidence showing that a horse can transmit flu to a human, or vice versa.

Q: How often does my horse need to be vaccinated?

A: We recommend yearly vaccinations to maintain a protective immunity. Some performance and show horses may need boosters four times a year.

Q: My horse was exposed to flu (rhino). Will he catch it?

A: If your horse has been vaccinated against flu (rhino), he should be protected, but we recommend a booster vaccination in cases of direct exposure. If your horse has never been vaccinated, you should have him vaccinated immediately as this will offer the best chance for resisting the disease.

Q: My mare is pregnant. Does she need any special vaccinations?

A: There is a form of rhino that infects the pregnant uterus. The doctor recommends giving rhino shots at the fifth, seventh, and ninth months of pregnancy to avoid a premature birth.

Q: My horse stepped on a nail. Does he need any shots?

A: Because the bacteria that cause tetanus can enter a horse's system through a puncture wound, your horse should get a tetanus antitoxin. This gives your horse immediate protection against tetanus.

Internal Parasite Questions

Q: What is a parasite?

A: A parasite is an organism that lives at the expense of another living being. In horses, this usually refers to intestinal worms.

Q: Why is parasite control important?

A: In horses, parasites are a major cause of poor

health. If left unchecked, they can cause serious, life-threatening problems.

Q: How can I control parasites?
A: It's very important to change pastures regularly and to feed out of buckets rather than off the ground. The doctor can help you establish a schedule of routine dewormings with alternating medicines.

Q: How can I tell if my horse has worms?
A: Bring a stool sample to the clinic, and the doctor will examine it for worms under a microscope. This is called a fecal exam.

Q: How often should my horse be checked?
A: Each situation is different, but normally once a year.

Q: My horse has bloodworms. Is that dangerous?
A: Bloodworms are very dangerous. If left untreated, bloodworms can cause severe damage to the horse's blood vessels and can even cause colic.

Q: My horse has little yellow specks on its lower legs. What are these, and what should I do about them?
A: The little yellow specks you're seeing are eggs layed by the adult bot fly. Bots are commonly seen in horses and can be treated with worm medicine.

Q: Can I get worms from my horse?
A: Under normal sanitary conditions, no.

Q: One of my horses has worms. Will the other horses get them?
A: If they share a pasture, it is very likely that one horse could infect the others. The doctor recommends treating the infected horse and checking a stool sample before it gets near your other horses.

Q: Can my horse get ringworm?
A: Yes. Ringworm is a fungal infection, not an actual worm. Horses are susceptible to this fungus just as dogs, cats, and humans are. It is treated with antifungal medication.

Q: My horse has been colicking a lot lately. Could this have anything to do with worms?
A: Colic is often a side effect of worm infestation. You should have a stool sample checked and get your horse on a regular deworming program if it is not already on one.

Q: Which is more effective, paste deworming or tube deworming?
A: Both methods are effective as long as they are done on a regular basis. If you're giving paste wormer at home, it's important to be sure that the horse is swallowing all the medicine.

Q: My horse has diarrhea. Does that mean it has worms?
A: Worms can often cause diarrhea, and we recommend a stool check and physical exam to determine what the problem is.

Other Parasite Questions

Reproduction Questions

Q: How often do mares come in heat?
A: Horses begin their heat cycles in early spring through summer. The longer amount of daylight stimulates this cycle. This is why most stud farms use artificial light.

Q: At what point in the heat cycle do I breed my mare?
A: When the mare stands for the stud. This normally means there is a large egg-containing follicle about to ovulate.

Q: At what age can I breed my mare?
A: The recommended age is usually 3.

Q: How long will my mare stay pregnant?
A: The gestation period is approximately 11 months.

Q: How can I tell when my mare is ready to deliver?
A: The mare will develop mammary tissue fullness (often referred to as being "bagged up"), and a small amount of yellow liquid will gel on the end of the teats. This is called waxing. When the wax falls off, the mare is very close to delivery.

Q: Will she need any help, or can she deliver the foal alone?
A: Normally mares deliver with no help. However, once the wax drops, they should be checked hourly.

Q: How long should the birth process take?
A: The normal delivery time in horses is about 30 minutes.

Q: Does my mare need any special attention or vaccinations while she's pregnant?

A: The doctor recommends giving rhinopneumonitis shots at five, seven, and nine months during pregnancy to prevent premature delivery.

Q: Should I have my male horse neutered?

A: Neutering, or gelding, will help prevent your horse from becoming overly aggressive, from fighting with other horses, and from exhibiting obnoxious sexual behavior. If you do not plan to use him for breeding, we highly recommend it.

Q: At what age should I have my male gelded?

A: It varies, but usually at about 18 months.

Q: Will gelding make my male horse fat and lazy?

A: No. If you watch his diet and give him plenty of exercise, there should be only natural weight gain.

Q: My horse has become aggressive and hard to handle. Will gelding him help reduce this?

A: Gelding has been shown to help reduce aggressiveness.

Q: Couldn't my horse just be given a vasectomy? Why does he have to be gelded?

A: Although it makes your horse incapable of breeding, a vasectomy does nothing to diminish his sexual drive and aggressiveness. By gelding, you reduce the hormones that are causing undesirable behavior.

Q: How old does my stallion have to be to be used for stud?

A: The length of time it takes for horses to reach sexual maturity varies. Generally a horse that is 2 1/2 years old is ready to be used for stud.

Q: Is artificial insemination used with horses, and is it safer than natural breeding?

A: Artificial breeding is used in the horse industry, but certain breeds require live coverage of the mare because the breed registry won't accept an artificially inseminated colt. With artificial breeding, there is less chance of injury.

Other Reproduction Questions

Medical Questions

Q: How do you take a horse's temperature?
A: By using a standard or digital lubricated rectal thermometer for three minutes (or until the digital thermometer signals the recoding is complete).

Q: What is a horse's normal temperature?
A: About 100 degrees Fahrenheit.

Q: What is a Coggins test, and why does my horse need one?
A: A Coggins test is a blood test that detects equine infectious anemia (EIA), a disease that is spread by insects. If a horse tests positive, it must be quarantined.

Q: If my horse gets EIA, can it be cured?
A: To date, there is no cure for this viral disease.

Q: What are wolf teeth?
A: Wolf teeth are small teeth in front of the molars, which may interfere with the bit. Some owners choose to have these teeth removed.

Q: A lot of grain falls out of my horse's mouth when he eats. What is causing this, and what should I do about it?
A: Your horse's teeth may need to be floated, or smoothed down, so that his chewing surface is flatter. Sharp points on molars can cause pain in a horse's mouth, which often gives him problems while he's chewing.

Q: What should I feed my horse? How often should she be fed?
A: Your horse should be fed grain (sweet feed or oats), hay, and water. How much to feed will depend on the amount of exercise the horse gets. Generally the horse should be fed enough to maintain its weight. Feedings should be divided into two or three portions throughout the day.

Q: Why is hay important?
A: The horse needs roughage in its diet to provide nutrients and for optimal digestion. This may be in the form of grass if a horse is in a pasture or hay if the horse is kept in a stall.

Q: My horse shakes its head a lot and seems sensitive around its ears. What causes this?
A: This usually indicates an irritation of the ear canal. This may be caused by ear ticks or a sensitivity to flies or gnats.

Q: My horse's eyes have been tearing a lot. Should I be worried about this?
A: Eye problems in horses should always be taken seriously and should be checked by the doctor as

soon as possible.

Q: I've heard a lot about colic. What is it, and how will I know if my horse has it?

A: Colic is acute abdominal pain, or a bad stomach ache. If your horse seems uncomfortable, stretches out, turns and looks at its stomach, or lies down and rolls and is reluctant to get up, you should call the doctor. Colic is serious. Horses with colic may have a mild, uncomplicated condition or a life-threatening intestinal blockage. The earlier colic is recognized and treated, the better the horse's chances are for recovery. Don't wait to see if the horse feels better in a while. If you suspect colic, call immediately.

Q: My gelding stretches out to urinate, but nothing comes out. What causes this, and what should I do about it?

A: This is a sign of pain and should be checked by the doctor as soon as possible.

Q: Should I put shoes on my horse? Will it hurt his feet or help keep them in better shape?

A: Shoes on horses are optional. They are for the protection of the horse's feet. Where the horse is being ridden and/or kept are deciding factors in whether to shoe your horse.

Q: What is founder?

A: Founder, or laminitis, is a severe inflammation of the feet. If you ever notice your horse reluctant to put weight on its front feet or acting like it's walking on eggs, call the doctor immediately—this is an emergency.

Q: Can founder be prevented?

A: Most of the time, founder is a result of bad

management, either overriding (road founder), or overeating. These types of founder can be avoided. However, founder that results from a severe illness is unpredictable and almost impossible to prevent.

Q: Can founder be cured?

A: Founder is a very serious condition. The earlier and more intense the treatment, the better the prognosis.

Other Medical Questions

Notes

Appendices

Glossary of Veterinary Medical Terms

A

abdomen: Portion of the body lying between the thorax and pelvis. The abdominal cavity contains the peritoneal cavity and its linings and the internal viscera.

aberration: Deviation from the normal condition.

abnormal: Not normal; deviation from the usual structure or condition.

abort: To miscarry or give birth prematurely before the fetus is developed enough to survive on its own.

abscess: Cavity filled with pus.

acute: Of sudden onset; having a short course.

aden/o-: Combining form for a gland or glandular.

adhesion: Abnormal fibrous union of tissues.

adipose: Fat; fatty.

adrenal gland: Paired glands, located near the kidneys, that produce various hormones, such as epinephrine and cortisol.

aerobic: Able to survive only in the presence of oxygen.

afterbirth: The placenta and associated membranes that are expelled from the uterus after the birth of the fetus.

albinism: Congenital lack of pigmentation (color) of the skin, eyes, and hair. An *albino* is an animal with albinism.

albumin: A major protein of blood plasma that is produced in the liver.

-algia: Word termination denoting pain or a painful condition.

alimentary: Pertaining to food or nutrient, or to the digestive system.

allergy: Hypersensitivity acquired through exposure to a particular substance (allergen).

alopecia: Loss of hair from an area in which hair is normally present.

ambi-: Prefix meaning both sides.

ambulate: To walk.

anaerobic: Able to survive only in the absence of oxygen.

analgesic: Capable of relieving pain; agent that reduces or eliminates pain but does not cause loss of consciousness.

*The glossary is abstracted in part from Phillip E. Cochran, *Guide to Veterinary Medical Terminology*. For more detailed definitions please refer to that work.

anatomy: Study of body structures and their positional relationships to each other.
andr/o-: Combining form meaning male.
anemia: Condition characterized by a lower-than-normal red blood cell count.
anesthesia: State of being without sensation, especially to pain. May or may not be accompanied by unconsciousness (general anesthesia vs. local anesthesia).
anesthetic: Agent that produces anesthesia, thus abolishing pain.
anestrus: Period of sexual inactivity between two estrous periods.
aneurysm: Dilation or outpouching of the wall of an artery, a vein, or the heart.
angi/o-: Combining form for a vessel. Usually refers to a blood vessel but may also refer to a lymph vessel.
anomaly: Marked deviation from normal.
anorexia: Lack of appetite.
anterior: Pertaining to the front of the body.
anthelmintic: Drug destructive to worms.
anti-: Prefix meaning against.
antibiotic: Drug used to kill bacteria and other microorganisms.
antibody: Protein in the body for specific protection against an allergen, invading organism, or foreign substance.
anticoagulant: Agent that prevents blood clotting.
anticonvulsant: Agent that prevents or stops convulsions.
antidiarrheal: Agent that combats diarrhea.
antidote: Agent used to counteract poison.
antiemetic: Agent that combats nausea and vomiting.
antifungal: Agent that inhibits or kills fungi.
antigen: Any substance that induces an immune response (antibody formation) by the body.
antihistamine: Agent that combats the effects of histamine.
anti-inflammatory: Agent that suppresses inflammation.
antipruritic: Agent that prevents or reduces itchiness.
antipyretic: Agent that reduces fever.
antitoxin: Antibody produced in response to exposure to a toxin produced by microorganisms, insects, or plants.
antitussive: Agent that combats coughing.
anus: Terminal opening or orifice of the alimentary canal (digestive tract).
aorta: Main trunk of the arterial system, originating from the

left side of the heart.

aperture: An opening or orifice.

appendage: Part attached to the main portion of an organ or the body, such as a limb or ear.

arrhythmia: Variation in rhythm of the heart.

arteri/o-: Combining form for artery.

artery: Vessel through which blood flows away from the heart to various parts of the body.

arthr/o-: Combining form for joint.

arthritis: Inflammation of a joint.

asepsis: Lack of infection or contamination by microorganisms.

aspirate: To remove fluid or gas from a cavity by suction; to inhale.

asthma: A condition involving the bronchial tree, in which the bronchi narrow, causing wheezing and hard breathing.

asymptomatic: Showing no signs of disease.

atrophy: Wasting away of a part.

atypical: Unusual; deviating from normal.

auditory: Pertaining to hearing.

autoclave: Machine that sterilizes medical instruments and materials by use of steam under pressure.

autopsy: Examination of a body after death.

avian: Pertaining to birds.

B

bacteria: A one-celled microorganism that may or may not cause disease.

balling gun: Device for administration of large tablets (boluses) to large animals.

barium: An element that is radiopaque (cannot be penetrated by X-rays). Used in diagnostic radiography.

benign: Not malignant; with a favorable prognosis.

bilateral: Occurring on two sides.

bile: Fluid that aids in digestion; produced in the liver and stored in the gall bladder.

biological: Medicine prepared from living organisms and their products, including sera, vaccines, antitoxins, antigens, bacterins, and toxoids.

biopsy: Removal of a small amount of tissue from the body for

examination, usually microscopic.
bitch: A female dog.
bladder: A sac serving as a receptacle for a secretion or excretion. Used alone, it refers to the urinary bladder.
bloat: Accumulation of gas in the stomach; a serious condition in dogs.
blood: Fluid, composed of water, cells, clotting factors, and other chemicals, that circulates through arteries, capillaries, and veins to supply nutrients and remove waste from tissues.
bloodworms: Worms of the class Nematoda, genus *Strongylus*. Specifically refers to *Strongylus vulgaris* found in horses.
bovine: Pertaining to cattle.
breech: Presentation of the fetal buttocks and tail in the birth canal during labor, with the hind limbs retained or extended beneath the fetal body.
brindle: Haircoat color pattern characterized by dark streaks or spots intermixed with brown, tan, or white hair.
bronchitis: Inflammation of the bronchi.
bronchus, bronchi: A large air passage in the lungs.

C

calculus, calculi: A stone or concretion formed inside the body, usually composed of mineral salts.
calf: A young bovine, less than a year old.
calve: To give birth to a calf.
cancer: A malignant tumor.
canine: Pertaining to dogs.
canine tooth: Large fang in carnivores.
cannon bone: The third metacarpal bone in the front leg of a horse.
capillary: Minute vessels connecting arterioles to venules, forming a network in almost all of the tissues of the body.
carcinoma: An invasive malignant tumor arising from epithelial tissues.
cardiac: Pertaining to the heart.
cardiopathy: Any disease of the heart.
carditis: Inflammation of the heart.
carnivore: Animal that eats flesh or meat.
cast: A stiff dressing or bandage used to immobilize a body part.
castrate: Surgical neutering of the male, which involves the

removal of both testicles.

cataract: Opacity of the lens of the eye.

catheter: A tubular instrument used to withdraw fluid from the body (such as urine), or to administer fluids, such as into a vein.

centesis: Perforation or tapping a body cavity or organ using a needle, aspirator, or trocar.

centi-: Prefix denoting one one-hundredth (1/100) of a unit.

centigrade: The Celsius temperature scale.

centimeter: 1/100 of a meter.

centrifuge: Machine that spins solutions at very high speeds so as to separate the lighter portions from the heavier portions.

cephalic: Pertaining to the head or head end of the body.

cerebellum: Part of the brain that coordinates movement.

cerebrum: The main portion of the brain that functions in thought, memory, and movement.

cerumen: Earwax.

chemotherapy: Treatment of disease, especially cancer, with chemical agents.

Chlamydia: A bacterium-like microorganism that is pathogenic to numerous domestic species of animals.

chlor/o-: Prefix meaning green.

choke: Obstruction of the esophagus, caused by a foreign body, food, or a stricture.

chronic: Persisting over a long period.

clot: A semisolid mass, as of blood cells.

coagulation: Clot formation.

coccus, cocci: A spherical bacterium.

coccyx: Group of vertebrae of the tail.

coffin bone: The main weight-bearing bone inside the horse's hoof.

colic: Acute abdominal pain; pertaining to the colon.

colitis: Inflammation of the colon.

colt: An intact male horse under 4 years old.

computerized axial tomography (CAT) scan; computed tomography (CT) scan: A technique that uses a special X-ray tube to obtain multiple images of an area of the body. Helps identify abnormalties that may not show up on a regualr X-ray.

conformation: The shape and arrangement of parts.

congenital: Present at birth.

conjunctiv/o-: The combining form for conjunctiva.
conjunctiva: Membrane that lines the inner eyelids and covers the exposed surface of the eyeball.
contra-: Prefix meaning against, opposed, or opposite of.
contraindication: A circumstance, condition, or disease that renders a particular treatment inappropriate or undesirable.
convulsion: Violent, involuntary contraction of skeletal muscles, originating from a neurological disorder.
copulation: Sexual union.
cornea: The transparent anterior portion of the fibrous outer tunic of the eye.
cortisone: A major hormone produced by the adrenal gland.
crani/o-: Combining form for the cranium or skull.
cranium: The skeleton of the head; the skull.
cryo-: Prefix relating to cold.
crypt/o-: Prefix meaning hidden or concealed.
cryptorchid: Male in which one or both testes have not descended into the scrotum.
C-section: The surgical delivery of a term fetus.
culture: A growth of microorganisms on living tissue cells or an artificial medium.
cure: Successful treatment of a disease, condition, or wound; the method used to treat the disease, condition, or wound.
cyanosis: Bluish discoloration of the mucous membranes and skin caused by poor tissue oxygenation.
cyst/o-: Combining form for bladder, usually the urinary bladder.
cystitis: Inflammation (by infection) of the urinary bladder.
cytology: Study of cells.
cytometer: Device used to count cells.

D

debride: To surgically remove foreign matter and devitalized tissues from a wound.
declaw: The surgical removal in cats of the nails and the nailbed so they do not grow back.
decongestant: Agent that reduces swelling or congestion of tissue.
defecation: Natural evacuation of fecal material from the rectum.
dehydration: Condition caused by excessive loss of water from

the body.
derma-: Combining form for skin.
dermatitis: Inflammation of the skin.
dermatology: Study of the skin and its disorders.
dermatosis: Any disease of the skin.
dewclaw: The first nonweight-bearing digit. The "thumb" of dogs and cats.
diagnosis: The documented cause of a disease or condition.
diarrhea: Abnormal liquidity of the feces and/or increased frequency of defecation.
dilation: Action of stretching to make bigger.
disease: Illness; deviation from normal physiologic function.
distal: Farthest from the central axis of the body.
diuresis: Increased production of urine.
diuretic: Agent that increases production of urine.
dock: Surgical removal of all or part of the tail of an animal.
dorsal: Pertaining to the back.
dose: A specified amount of medication or other therapeutic agent.
dosimetry: Determination of the amount of radiation emanating from a source.
duodenum: the portion of the small intestine just below the stomach.
drug: Any substance used to prevent, diagnose, or treat disease.
dwarf: Abnormally small or undersized animal.
dys-: Prefix meaning difficult, painful, or impaired.
dysfunction: Impaired or abnormal function.
dysplasia: See hip dysplasia.

E

ect/o-: Prefix meaning outside, outer, or on the outer part.
-ectomy: Suffix meaning excision of an organ part.
ectoparasite: Plant or animal that lives on the skin or in external openings of its host.
edema: A swelling of tissue caused by excessive fluid retention.
electrocardiogram (ECG): Tracing produced by electrical impulses associated with contraction of the heart muscle.
electrocardiograph: Instrument used to record the ECG.
electroencephalography (EEG): Procedure of recording the electrical currents produced by the brain.

Elizabethan collar: Funnel-shaped sheet of cardboard, plastic, or X-ray film placed around an animal's neck to prevent it from chewing itself.
emaciation: State of extreme weight loss.
emasculator: Instrument used to castrate a large animal.
embolism: Sudden obstruction of a blood vessel by a clot or foreign material brought to the area by the flow of blood.
emesis: Act of vomiting.
-emia: Suffix relating to blood.
encephal/o-: Combining form for the brain.
encephalitis: Inflammation of the brain.
end/o-: Prefix meaning inward or inside.
endocarditis: Inflammation of the lining of the heart chambers.
endocrine: Relating to ductless glands that secrete hormones into the blood stream.
endometrium: Lining of the uterus.
endoparasite: Animal that lives within its host.
endotracheal tube: Flexible tube placed into the trachea through the mouth to administer inhalant gases.
enema: Liquid injected into the rectum to stimulate bowel movement.
entrails: Internal organs of animals.
enucleation: Surgical removal of the eye.
epidermis: The most superficial nonvascular layer of the skin.
epiglottis: Lip-like cartilaginous structure that covers the opening to the larynx during swallowing.
epilepsy: A disease of the brain characterized by periodic seizure activity or loss of consciousness.
equine: Pertaining to horses.
ehrlichiosis: A disease of dogs transmitted by ticks and often manifested by a nosebleed.
erythrocyte: Red blood cell.
esophagus: Anatomical tube that connects the mouth to the stomach.
estrus: The portion of the heat cycle during which the female is ready to breed.
euthanasia: The painless inducement of death, usually by intravenous injection.
exacerbation: Increase in severity or clinical signs of a disease or condition.

excise: To cut out or off; to remove surgically.
excretion: Act of removing or discharging products from the body, such as urine or perspiration.
exhale: To expel from the lungs by breathing.
extension: Movement in which a flexed limb is straightened.
extra-: Prefix meaning outside of, beyond, or in addition to.

F

fallopian tube: Tube connecting the ovary and uterus, through which ova are transported.
febrile: Characterized by fever.
feces: Waste products discharged from the intestinal tract.
feline: Pertaining to cats.
femoral: Pertaining to the femur or thigh.
femur: Bone extending from the pelvis to the knee; the thigh bone.
fetlock joint: Leg joint in the horse.
filly: Young female horse up to 4 years old or until the animal is first bred.
flank: Lateral part of the animal's body extending from the ribs to the ileum.
flexion: Act of bending.
float: To file off the sharp edges from a horse's teeth; device used to do the filing.
foal: Process of giving birth in horses; horse less than 1 year of age.
footrot: Necrosis of the hoof caused by infection.
forelock: Lock of hair lying on the forehead of a horse.
founder: Inflammation of the sensitive structures of the foot in hoofed animals; laminitis.
fracture: The breaking of a bone.
friable: Easily torn or crumbled.
frog: A V-shaped band or horny tissue on the under-surface of a horse's hoof.
fungus: Plant without chlorophyll, such as molds, yeasts, and ringworm.
fur ball: A hairball.

G

gait: Manner of walking, running, or moving.
gallbladder: Reservoir for bile located near the liver.
gaskin: Area of the hind leg extending from knee to hock.
gastr/o-: Combining form for stomach.
gastritis: Inflammation of the stomach.
gastroenterology: Study of disorders of the stomach and intestines.
geld: Act of castrating a male horse.
gelding: A castrated male horse.
generic: Referring to a drug name not protected by a trademark.
genital: Pertaining to reproduction or the reproductive organs.
genitalia: The reproductive organs.
geriatrics: Branch of medicine dealing with old and aging animals.
gestation: Period of pregnancy.
giant: Animal, person, or organism of enormous size.
gingiva: The gums.
glottis: The opening between the vocal cords.
gonad: The ovary in females or testes in males.
graft: Any tissue or organ transplanted to or implanted at another location on the body or another body.
-gram: Suffix meaning a written record or image.
gram: 1/1000 of a kilogram.
granulation: Formation of a small, round, red, fleshy mass in wounds.
-graph: Suffix referring to an instrument for writing or recording.
grave: Very serious or severe.
gum: Common name for gingiva.

H

hairball: Loose clump of hair (or fur), food, and other debris in the stomach.
heart: Muscular organ in the chest that pumps the blood throughout the body.
heat: Common name for estrus.
hem/o, hema-, hemat/o-: Combining forms for blood.
hemacytometer: Electronic instrument or calibrated glass chamber used to count blood cells.
hematocrit: Packed cell volume; volume percentage of red blood

cells in whole blood.

hematology: Study of blood.

hematoma: Localized collection of blood in an organ, space, or tissue; in dogs and cats, usually seen in the ear.

hemoglobin: The oxygen-carrying pigment of red blood cells.

hemorrhage: Escape of blood from a vessel; bleeding.

hemostasis: Arrest of bleeding.

hemostat: Instrument used to clamp blood vessels to stop bleeding.

hepat/o-: Combining form for liver.

hepatosis: Any disorder of the liver.

hernia: Protrusion of an organ or tissue through an abdominal opening.

heter/o-: Prefix meaning other or another.

heterosexual: Pertaining to the opposite sex; preferring the opposite sex.

hip dysplasia: Malformation of the hip joint; can lead to arthritis.

hist/o-: Combining form for tissue.

histamine: Naturally occurring substance found in all body tissues that is a component of the inflammatory reaction.

histology: Study of tissues at the microscopic level.

histopathology: Study of diseased tissues at the microscopic level.

hives: Raised, red patches of skin, often accompanied by itchiness.

hock: The joint distal to the knee in the rear leg.

homeo-: Prefix meaning alike.

homeostasis: Stability of the normal physiologic state.

homo-: Prefix meaning the same.

hoof knife: Instrument used to pare away horny tissue from a hoof.

hormone: Substance produced by an organ causing a specific effect on other organs or tissues.

host: Animal or plant that harbors a parasite, providing it with nourishment.

hydrotherapy: Use of water in treatment of disease.

hyper-: Prefix meaning excessive, abnormally high.

hypertension: High blood pressure.

hyperthermia: High body temperature.

hypo-: Prefix meaning deficient, abnormally low.

hypotension: Low blood pressure.
hypothermia: Low body temperature.
hyster/o-: Combining form for uterus.
hysterectomy: Excision of the uterus.

I

-ia: Suffix indicating state or condition.
-iasis: Suffix meaning a process or condition resulting therefrom.
icterus: Yellow discolorations of the skin and mucous membranes caused by bile pigments; jaundice.
idiopathic: Of unknown cause.
immune: Highly resistant to disease because of formation of antibodies.
inbreeding: Mating of closely related animals with similar genetic constitutions.
incise: To cut.
incision: Wound produced by a sharp instrument.
incisor: Blade-like front tooth adapted for cutting.
incontinent: Unable to control urination or defecation.
incubation: Development of microorganisms in a host or culture medium.
incubation period: The amount of time from contact with a disease-producing organism until the disease manifests itself.
incubator: Environmentally controlled chamber for incubation of cultures, eggs, or living cells, or treatment of newborn or sick animals.
infection: Invasion of the body by microorganisms.
infectious: Capable of causing infection, or caused by or capable of being transmitted by infection.
inflammation: Localized tissue response to injury, characterized by heat, swelling, redness, pain, and loss of function.
influenza: Acute viral respiratory infection; flu.
infra-: Prefix meaning below or beneath.
inhale: To take into the lungs by breathing.
injection: Introduction of a fluid, by force, into a vessel or part.
insecticide: A chemical used to kill insects.
intact: State of being sexually whole and not spayed or castrated.
inter-: Prefix meaning between.
internal medicine: Specialty dealing with disorders of the internal body systems.

intestine: Portion of the digestive tract; also called the bowel.
intra-: Prefix meaning within.
intramuscular: Within a muscle.
intravenous: Within a vein.
intubate: To insert a tube into a body canal or hollow organ, such as the trachea or stomach.
iris: Colored membrane in the eye; surrounds the pupil.
irradiation: Treatment or exposure to radiation.
irrigate: To wash out or flush.
-ism: Suffix meaning a state or condition.
-itis: Suffix denoting inflammation.

J

jaundice: Yellow discoloration of the skin and mucous membranes caused by bile; common in severe liver disorders.
joint: Junction between bones.
juvenile: Pertaining to youth or immaturity.

K

keratitis: Inflammation of the cornea.
kidney: A paired organ that filters waste products from the blood to produce urine.
kilo-: Prefix indicating 1,000.
kilogram: 1,000 grams; 2.2 pounds.

L

laceration: A wound made by tearing or cutting.
lacrimal: Pertaining to tears.
laminitis: Inflammation of the sensitive structures of the foot in hoofed animals; founder.
lance: To cut open with a pointed knife or scalpel.
laryng/o-: Combining form for larynx.
larynx: Structure containing the vocal cords.
lateral: Pertaining to the side of the body.
lesion: Any discontinuity of tissue or loss of function.
lethal: Deadly or fatal.
leuk/o-: Prefix relating to white blood cells.
leukemia: Malignant disease of the blood.
leukocyte: A white blood cell.

ligament: Band of dense, fibrous tissue connecting bones and supporting joints.
ligate: To tie off.
ligature: Material used to tie off a vessel.
lingual: Pertaining to the tongue.
lip/o-: Combining form for fat.
lipoma: Benign tumor composed of fat cells.
liter: 1,000 milliliters, approximately 1 quart.
litter: Numerous young born at one time of the same mother.
liver: Large gland responsible for numerous critical metabolic functions.
lockjaw: Common name for tetanus.
lumbar: Part of the back between the chest and pelvis.
lung: Organ of respiration located in the chest cavity.
luxation: Dislocation.
lymph: Transparent, whitish-yellow liquid derived from tissue fluids.
lymphatic: Pertaining to a lymph vessel.
-lysis: Destruction of cells.

M

macro-: Prefix meaning large.
magnetic resonance imaging (MRI): A technique that uses a magnetic field to produce two-dimensional images of internal organs or structures. Provides better visualization of soft tissues than X-rays and more view angles than a CT scan.
mal-: Prefix meaning bad, diseased, or impaired.
malignant: Tending to become progressively worse and result in death. Often refers to potentially fatal tumors.
malocclusion: Improper alignment of the teeth.
malpresentation: Abnormal presentation of the fetus in the birth canal.
mamm/o-: Combining form for mammary glands.
mammal: A warm-blooded vertebrate that has hair and suckles its young.
mammary glands: Female glandular structures that secrete milk.
mammography: Radiography of the mammary glands.
mandible: The lower jaw bone.
mane: The long hair growing on the top of a horse's neck from

head to withers.

marrow: Soft, jelly-like material that fills the cavities of bones; a site of blood cell formation.

mast/o-: Combining form for mammary glands.

mastectomy: Excision of mammary tissue.

mastitis: Inflammation of the mammary glands.

maxilla: Skull bone forming the upper jaw.

medial: Denoting a position toward the middle of the body.

median: Vertical midline of the body.

medicine: Any drug or remedy; the art or science of treating disease by nonsurgical means.

medium: Nutritive substance used in the culture of microorganisms.

medulla: Inner portion of an organ or structure.

mega-: Prefix meaning of great size or enlarged.

megacolon: An abnormally enlarged colon.

-megaly: Suffix meaning abnormally large.

melan/o-: Prefix meaning black or relating to melanin, a dark body pigment, found in skin, hair, some tumors, the eye, and other tissues.

melanoma: Tumor comprised of cells containing melanin.

meningitis: Inflammation of the membranes enveloping the brain or spinal cord.

mes/o-: Prefix meaning middle or intermediate.

metabolic: Pertaining to the processes by which cells and tissues are produced and maintained.

metastasis: Transfer of disease from one organ or area of the body to another; usually refers to the spread of tumor cells.

meter: 1,000 millimeters or approximately 39.37 inches; instrument used in measuring.

micro-: Prefix designating small size.

microbiology: Study of microorganisms, such as bacteria, viruses, and fungi.

microorganism: Minute (usually microscopic) living organism, such as viruses, bacteria, fungi, and protozoa.

microscope: Instrument used to view minute objects in detail not possible to see with the naked eye.

milliliter: 1/1,000 of a liter, abbreviated ml.

mon/o-: Prefix meaning one or single.

morbid: Unhealthy; diseased.

morbidity: Ratio of sick to healthy animals in a population.
moribund: Dying; near death.
morphology: Study of form and structure of organisms; form and structure of an organism.
mortality: Death rate; ratio of total deaths in a given population.
motor: Producing movement.
mucosa: Membrane lining tubular organ such as the alimentary tract; a mucous membrane.
mucous: Pertaining to or resembling mucus; secreting mucus.
mucus: The slimy secretion found on mucous membranes.
multi-: Prefix meaning many.
muscle: Tissue with the ability to contract.
muzzle: The nose and upper and lower mouth; a device placed around the snout and jaw to prevent biting.
my/o-: Combining form for muscle.
myocardium: The muscular layer of the heart wall.

N

nape: The back of the neck.
narc/o-: Combining form meaning stupor or stuporous.
narcotic: Pertaining to or producing stupor or insensibility; agent that produces stupor.
naris, nares: Moist opening of the nasal cavity, the nostril.
natal, -natal: Pertaining to birth.
navicular: Pertaining to the navicular bone in the horse, which lies near the coffin bone.
necr/o-: Prefix relating to death or dead tissue.
necropsy: Examination of a body after death. *Necropsy* is the preferred term for examination of animal cadavers, *autopsy* for humans.
necrosis: Death of tissue.
necrotic: Pertaining to dead tissue.
neo-: Prefix meaning new or strange.
neonatal: Pertaining to the first few weeks after birth.
neoplasm: Any new or abnormal growth, especially one which is progressive and uncontrolled; a tumor.
nephr/o-: Combining form for kidney.
nephrosis: Any disease of the kidney.
nerve: Cord-like structure, made up of numerous fibers, that carries impulses between the central nervous system and

some other part of the body.
neuro-: Combining form for nerve.
neurology: Study of the brain, spinal cord, and nerves.
neuter: To surgically remove the reproductive organs in either the male (castration) or female (spay).

O

occipital: Pertaining to the area of the back of the head.
occlusion: The act of closing off; an obstruction.
ocul/o-: Combining form for eye.
odont/o-: Combining form for teeth.
oncologist: Specialist in tumors.
oncology: Study of tumors.
operation: Surgical procedure.
ophthalm/o-: Combining form for eye.
ophthalmic: Pertaining to the eye; medication used in the eye.
ophthalmology: Study of disorders of the eye.
-opia: Suffix relating to vision.
orifice: The opening, entrance, or outlet of a body cavity.
orthopedic: Pertaining to bones and the skeletal system.
-osis: Suffix meaning a disease.
oste/o-: Combining form for bone.
ot/o-: Combining form for ear.
otic: Pertaining to the ear; medication used in the ear.
otoscope: Instrument used to view the external ear canal and the tympanic membrane.
ovari/o-: Combining form for ovaries.
ovariectomy: Surgical removal of one or both ovaries.
ovariohysterectomy: Surgical removal of the ovaries and uterus; spay.
ovary: The sexual gland of the female in which ova (or eggs) are formed.
oviduct: Tubular passage that carries ova to the uterus.
ovum, ova: The female reproductive cell, an egg.
-oxia: Suffix relating to oxygen.

P

palate: Partition separating the oral and nasal cavities.
palpation: Using the hands to feel body parts during physical

examination. Often refers to checking a mare for pregnancy.
pancreas: Gland that produces the digestive enzymes insulin and glucagon.
panleukopenia: Viral disease of cats characterized by decreased numbers of white blood cells.
papilloma: Benign skin tumor; wart.
paralysis: Loss or impairment of the ability to move body parts.
parameter: A measure of value of a body function.
paraplegia: Paralysis of both rear legs.
parasite: Plant or animal that lives on or in another organism at the expense of the host.
parasitology: Study of parasites.
parenteral: By a route of administration other than through the mouth (for example, intravenous or subcutaneous).
paresis: Slight or incomplete paralysis.
paroxysm: Sudden recurrence or intensification of sign; a spasm or seizure.
parturition: The act of giving birth.
pastern: Area of the horse's leg between the fetlock and the hoof.
path/o-: Prefix relating to disease.
pathogen: A disease-producing microorganism.
pathogenic: Causing disease.
pathologic: Indicating disease.
pathology: Study of the nature of disease, especially the effects of disease on tissue structure and function.
-pathy: Suffix meaning disease.
pediatrics: Branch of medicine dealing with young animals.
pelvis: The paired hip bones.
-penia: Suffix meaning a deficiency; subnormal numbers.
peri-: Prefix meaning around or near.
perianal: Located around the anus.
perinatal: Pertaining to the period shortly before and after birth.
periodontal: Pertaining to the area around a tooth.
peripheral: Situated away from the central area of the body.
peritoneal cavity: Space within the abdominal cavity between the viscera and the abdominal wall.
peritoneum: Serous membrane that lines the wall of the abdominal cavity and envelops the abdominal organs.
permeable: Permitting a substance to pass through.
Petri dish: Shallow glass or plastic dish for growing cultures

of microorganisms.
phag/o-: Prefix relating to eating.
phalanx: Toe.
pharmaceutical: Pertaining to drugs; a drug.
pharmacology: Study of drugs and their actions.
pharmacy: Science of preparing and dispensing drugs; area within a hospital where drugs are prepared and dispensed.
pharynx: Passage between the nostrils and the esophagus and larynx.
phleb/o-: Combining form for vein.
phlebitis: Inflammation of a vein.
phobia: Any excessive or unreasonable fear.
placenta: The membranes surrounding the developing fetus in mammals, providing nutrition.
-plasia: Suffix referring to development relative to numbers of cells.
-plegia: Suffix meaning paralysis.
pleura: Serous membrane that lines the thoracic (chest) cavity and envelops the thoracic organs.
pleural cavity: Space within the thoracic cavity between the thoracic organs and the body wall.
pneum/o-: Combining form relating to the lungs or breath.
pneumonia: Infection of the lungs.
poly-: Prefix meaning many.
polydactyly: Presence of extra toes.
post-: Prefix meaning after or behind.
postmortem: After death.
posterior: Pertaining to the rear or back part of the body.
postnasal: Situated or occurring behind the nose or nasal passage.
postoperative: Occurring after surgery.
practitioner: One who diagnoses and treats diseases.
pre-: Prefix meaning before.
preadult: Before maturity or before the adult period of life.
preoperative: Occurring before surgery.
prescription: Written direction for preparation and dosage of a drug.
pro-: Prefix meaning before or in front of.
proestrus: Period preceding estrus or heat.
prognosis: Forecast of the probable outcome of a disease.

prolapse: Protrusion, falling down, or sinking of an organ (or part of an organ), often through a normal body opening.
prone: Lying with the face down.
prophylaxis: Prevention of disease.
prostate: An accessory sex gland in some male animals.
prostatitis: Inflammation of the prostate gland.
pruritus: Itchiness.
pseud/o-: Combining form meaning false.
psych/o-: Combining form relating to the mind.
psychology: Branch of science dealing with mental processes, especially behavior.
psychomotor: Pertaining to brain activity resulting in movement.
puberty: Time at which an animal achieves sexual maturity and can reproduce.
pulm/o-: Combining form for the lungs.
purulent: Consisting of or containing pus.
pus: Liquid product of inflammation comprised of white blood cells, cellular debris, and other matter.
putrefaction: Decomposition by body enzymes that produces a foul smell.
pyo-: Prefix relating to pus.
pyometra: Accumulation of pus in the uterus.

Q

quad-, quadri-: Prefix meaning four.
quadruped: Animal with four feet.
queen: Process of giving birth in cats; an adult intact female cat.
quick: The sensitive tissues of the claw or hoof.

R

radi/o-: Combining form for radiation.
radiogram: Image on film produced by passage of X-rays through a body part.
radiograph: A radiogram.
radiography: The act of making a radiogram by use of an X-ray machine.
radiology: Study of the use of radiation in diagnosis and treatment of disease.
radiopaque: Not permitting passage of radiation.
radius: A bone between the elbow and carpal joint (wrist).

rectum: Distal portion of the large intestine, ending at the anus.
recumbent: Lying down.
refracture: To break a previously broken bone that was healed abnormally.
regurgitate: To vomit food that has not yet reached the stomach.
rehydrate: To replace lost body fluids.
relapse: Return of disease after apparent cure.
remission: Lessening of signs of a disease; the period when signs of disease have decreased.
ren/o-: Combining form for kidney.
resident: Graduate veterinarian (or physician) being trained in a specialty area in a hospital.
resistance: Natural ability of the body to remain unaffected by microorganisms and poisons.
resorb: To take up or absorb again.
respiration: The act of breathing.
restraint: Forcibly holding an animal or body part still during examination or treatment.
retina: The innermost layer of the eye, containing the cells that respond to light.
rheumatism: Condition characterized by inflammation or degeneration of joints.
rhin/o-: Combining form for nose.
rhinitis: Inflammation of the mucous membranes of the nasal passages.
rigor mortis: Stiffening of a dead body.
rump: Area around the point of the hips and tailhead.

S

sacr/o-: Combining form for sacrum.
sacrum: Portion of the lower spinal column.
saline: Salty; containing salts.
saliva: Clear secretion from the mucous glands of the mouth.
salivary: Pertaining to saliva.
sanguineous: Containing much blood.
sarcoid: Beginning skin tumor of horses.
sarcoma: Malignant tumor.
scalpel: Small surgical knife with a straight handle and usually a detachable blade.
scapula: Shoulder blade.

sclera: The tough, white, outer part of the eyeball.
sclerosis: Hardening of tissue, especially following inflammation.
-scope: Suffix meaning an instrument used for examining, viewing, listening, or detecting.
scrotum: The pouch containing the testes.
scruff: Common name for the loose skin around the neck and shoulders of dogs, cats, and other small animals.
sedative: Agent that reduces activity or decreases excitement.
seizure: A convulsion.
semen: The thick, whitish reproductive secretion of males.
semi-: Prefix meaning half or partially.
senile: Pertaining to old age.
sepsis: Presence of microorganisms or their toxins in the blood.
serum, sera: The liquid portion of the blood remaining after removal of the solid elements and blood cells.
shock: Acute circulatory failure characterized by hypotension, cool extremities, and rapid heart rate.
sign: Objective evidence of disease as perceived by the examining veterinarian.
sinus: Cavity or hollow space.
sinusitis: Inflammation of a paranasal sinus.
slough: To cast off or shed, especially dead tissue.
snout: The elongated nasal area of certain species, extending from the eyes to the nostrils.
sole: The undersurface of a foot or hoof.
soma: Pertaining to the body (used alone or as a prefix or suffix).
spasm: A sudden, violent, involuntary muscle contraction that is usually painful.
spay: See **ovariohysterectomy**.
specialist: Practitioner who concentrates on a particular branch of medicine or surgery.
specialty: Any particular branch of medicine.
species: Category in the classification of organisms.
spermatozoa: Mature male germ (reproductive) cells.
sphincter: Ring-like band of muscle that closes a natural body opening.
spinal: Pertaining to the vertebral column.
spleen: A large organ near the stomach that stores red blood cells.
splint: A rigid or flexible appliance used to stabilize or prevent

movement of a part.

sprain: Injury (but not rupture) of ligaments supporting a joint.

staphylococcus: A type of bacteria.

stasis, -stasis: Cessation of or reduced flow.

status: State or condition.

sterile: Free of microorganisms; unable to reproduce.

steroid: Compound in a group of chemicals, resembling cholesterol, that includes the sex hormones, glucocorticoids, mineralocorticoids, and bile acids.

stethoscope: Instrument used to listen to body sounds.

stifle: The "knee" of the rear leg.

stitch: Common term for a suture.

stomach: The expanded part of the alimentary canal between the esophagus and duodenum.

stomat/o-: Combining form for mouth.

stool: Feces.

streptococcus: A type of bacteria.

stupor: Partially unconscious.

sub-: Prefix meaning under, near, almost, or moderately.

subcutaneous: Beneath the skin.

subnormal: Below normal.

super-: Prefix meaning above or excess.

superficial: Near the surface.

supine: Lying face up.

supra-: Prefix meaning above or over.

surgeon: A doctor who performs surgeries.

surgery: A branch of medicine that treats disease by operative procedures; an operation; the place where operations are performed.

susceptible: Not immune.

suture: Material used to close a wound or tie off a bleeding vessel; the act of closing a wound or uniting two tissue surfaces.

symptom: Subjective evidence of disease as perceived by a human patient.

syndrome: A set of clinical signs occurring together as the usual course of a disease or condition.

syringe: Calibrated tubular instrument used for injecting or withdrawing liquids into or from the body.

systemic: Affecting the body as a whole.

T

tendon: A fibrous cord by which muscle is attached to bone or to other muscles.
tension: The act of stretching or being stretched or strained.
testicle: Testis; the male gonad.
testis, testes: The male gonad that produces spermatozoa and male hormones.
tetanus: Infectious disease caused by bacterial toxin, characterized by tonic muscular spasm; lockjaw.
tetra-: Combining form meaning four.
therapeutic: Pertaining to treatment or healing.
therapy: Treatment of disease.
therm/o-: Prefix relating to heat.
-thermia, -thermy: Suffixes relating to heat.
thermometer: Instrument for measuring temperatures.
thigh: Area of the rear leg between the hip and the stifle.
thoracic: Pertaining to the thorax.
thorax: The chest.
thromb/o-: Prefix relating to a clot.
thrombus, thrombi: A blood clot.
thrush: Common name for footrot or infection of the sole of the hoof in horses.
thyroid: Paired gland, located on either side of the trachea, that produces hormones regulating body metabolism.
tibia: The shin bone.
tic: An involuntary repetitive muscular contraction, usually of facial or shoulder muscles.
tick: An external parasite which feeds on the blood of its host.
tissue: An aggregation of cells specialized in one function.
-tomy: Suffix meaning to cut into or make an incision.
tonic: Characterized by continuous tension or state of contraction.
tonsil: A small, rounded mass of lymphoid tissue, located on both sides at the rear of the mouth (top of the throat).
tonsillectomy: Surgical removal of one or both tonsils.
tonsillitis: Inflammation of the tonsils.
topical: Pertaining to a surface area; often refers to medicines used on the outside of the body.
torsion: Twisting or rotation.
tourniquet: Any device applied to an extremity or part to reduce blood flow.

tox/o-, toxi-, toxic/o-: Prefixes relating to poisons.
toxemia: Condition resulting from bacterial toxins in the blood stream.
toxicology: Study of poisons.
toxin: A poison.
toxoid: A vaccine made of modified bacterial toxins, used to stimulate an immune response against toxins produced by those bacteria.
trachea: Tubular airway connecting the larynx to the bronchi.
tranquilizer: Drug used to calm an animal or relieve anxiety without necessarily altering consciousness or clarity of thought.
trans-: Prefix meaning across, through or beyond.
transfusion: Introduction of whole blood or blood components into the bloodstream.
transient: Temporary.
translucent: Transmitting light, but diffusing it so that the objects behind it are not clearly visible.
trauma: A wound or injury.
traumatic: Pertaining to or as a result of injury.
tri-: Prefix meaning three.
trimester: A period of three months; often used when referring to pregnancy.
tumor: A swelling or pathologic enlargement of tissues; a neoplasm.
turbid: Cloudy.
twitch: Device applied to the lip, ear, or another part of horses for restraint during minor procedures.
tympanic membrane: The eardrum.

U

ulcer: A local defect or excavation of the surface of an organ or tissue, caused by sloughing of dead tissue.
ultra-: Prefix meaning beyond or extreme.
umbilicus: The navel; the scar marking the site of the fetal umbilical cord.
un-: Prefix meaning not, opposite of.
uni-: Prefix meaning one or single.
unicellular: One-celled.
unilateral: Affecting only one side.

unsoundness: In horses, any disease, condition, or defect that causes lameness or an abnormal gait.
ur/o-: Combining form relating to urine, urination, or the urinary system.
ureter: The fibromuscular tube that conveys urine from each kidney to the bladder.
urethra: The tube that conveys urine from the bladder to the exterior of the body.
urinalysis: Analysis of urine by chemical and microscopic examination.
urination: Passage or discharge of urine.
urine: Fluid formed in the kidneys, passed to the bladder for storage, and discharged through the urethra.
urology: Study of disorders of the urinary system.
uterus: A hollow muscular organ, found in female mammals, in which the fertilized ovum develops.

V

vaccine: An agent that, when introduced into the body, stimulates an immune response against certain microorganisms.
vagina: The canal in females extending from the vulva to the cervix.
vas/o-: Combining form for vessels or ducts.
vein: Vessel through which blood returns from organs and body parts to the heart.
ven/o-: Combining form for vein.
venipuncture: Puncture of a vein with a needle.
ventilation: The process of exchanging air between the lungs and the atmosphere; the process of replacement of air in a room by mechanical means.
ventral: Pertaining to the belly or underside of a quadruped.
ventricle: A small cavity, such as the lower chambers of the heart.
venule: Very small vessels that collect blood from the capillaries, then join to form veins.
vertebrate: Any animal with a spinal column; having a spinal column.
vessel: Any channel, tube, or duct for carrying fluid, such as blood or lymph.

veterinarian: Doctor of veterinary medicine.
veterinary: Pertaining to domestic animals and their diseases.
viable: Capable of living; remaining alive.
virology: Study of viruses and the diseases they produce.
virulence: The degree to which a microorganism can cause serious disease.
virus: A minute infectious agent that replicates only inside a living cell and lacks the ability for independent metabolism.
viscous: Sticky or adhesive.
viscera: Any large organs located within the thoracic or abdominal cavities or within the pelvic canal.
vomit: To cast up material from the stomach.
vulva: External genitalia of females, including the labia and vaginal opening.

W

wall: The hard tissue making up the outer surface of a horse's hoof; the limiting tissue surrounding a cavity, such as the abdominal wall surrounding the abdominal cavity.
wean: To discontinue nursing or suckling a young animal.
weanling: Young animal recently changed from suckling to another source of food.
whelp: The process of giving birth in dogs.
withers: The top or highest point of the shoulders of horses or dogs.
Wood's light: An ultraviolet light, often used to detect ringworm on the skin of animals.
wound: Any disruption of the continuity of a normal structure, as from incision or injury.

X

X-ray: An electromagnetic vibration used to diagnose and treat disease.

Z

zoo-: Combining form relating to animals.
zoonosis: A disease of animals that can be transmitted to people under natural conditions.

VITAL STATISTICS*

Species	Normal temp. (°F)	Gestation period (days)	Litter size	Life span (yrs.)	Respiration (breaths/min.)	Heart rate (beats/min.)
Canine	101.5	63	varies	8-18 (varies)	22	100-130
Feline	101.5	63	varies	8-18 (varies)	26	110-140
Equine	100	340	1	16-20 (varies)	12	30 adult 60 colt
Ferret	100-102.5	42	6-10	8-14	NA	NA
Gerbil	100.8	24	1-12	4	NA	NA
Hamster	100	16	4-10	2-3	NA	NA
Rabbit	102	28-36	7	5-7	NA	NA

**All values are approximate and may vary from animal to animal.*

Index

A

Abscesses 184, 214, 230
Allergies 68, 96, 113, 152, 170, 183, 213-214
Anal gland impaction 178,199
Anesthesia 168-171, 231
Appointments
  dentistry 70
  duty schedules 66-68
  large-animal 76-77
  marketing ideas 62
  post-hospitalization care/discharge 97-100
  scheduling 65-77
  surgery 70-75
  SEE ALSO Client relations, Telephone policies
Asthma 180, 184, 232
Attire 35-36

B

Bad breath 179
Billing inquiries 21, 46-50
Bladder stones 127, 175
Bloating 93, 215, 233
Bloodworm 147, 149, 187, 220, 233
Body temperature 211, 224, 257
Bots 149, 220
Breeding SEE Heat cycles
Burial arrangements
  SEE Grief counseling

C

Canine diseases
  SEE Diseases, canine
Castration (neuter)
  dogs and cats 172-173, 208-209
  horses 223
Cesarean section 174
Choking 180
Client relations
  anxious owners 97
  client without an appointment 3-4
  emergency clinics 30-31, 84-87
  fee estimates 98-99
  grief counseling 100-103
  new clients 114-116
  unavoidable delays 5-6
  unhappy clients 104-110
  unruly clients 35
  SEE ALSO Appointments, Referrals, Telephone policies
Coccidia 140, 142
Coggins test 224
Colic 87, 93, 187, 221, 226, 234
Commonly asked questions
  horses 218-228
  small animals 192-216
Computer-enhanced images 128
Constipation, feline 185
Corneal ulcer 187
Coronavirus 132

D

Death of pet SEE Grief counseling
Declaw, feline 173, 235
Dentistry

appointments for 70
bad breath 179
equine 187, 225
gingivitis/tartar 179
Dewclaw removal 173-174
Diagnosis
by phone 38-43
tests/lab work 124-126
Diarrhea 93, 132, 140, 193, 199-200, 215, 221-222, 236
Diseases, canine
coronavirus 132
distemper 131, 192-195,
hepatitis 131
kennel cough 132, 212
leptospirosis 131
Lyme disease 132, 154, 195, 203
parvovirus 132, 193-195
rabies 132, 192-194
Diseases, equine
encephalomyelitis 134
influenza 135, 218-219
rhinopneumonitis 135, 219
strangles 136
tetanus 136, 219
Diseases, feline
distemper 133, 192-195
feline immunodeficiency virus (FIV) 196
feline infectious peritonitis (FIP) 125, 133
leukemia 125, 133-134, 195
rabies 134, 192-194
upper respiratory diseases 134
Distemper, canine 131, 192-195
Distemper, feline 133, 192-195
Dress code 35-36
Drugs 158-162
Drugs, nonprescription 118, 164-165
Drugs, prescription 158-164
abbreviations 166
dispensing 158-164
labeling 159-161
pharmacy 160-161

E

Ear problems 180
Electrolytes 125
Emergencies
after-hours 86-87
clinics 30-31, 84-87
common large animal emergencies 93-94
common small-animal emergencies 92-93
fees for 90-92
in-clinic 81-85
poison 83
procedures for 80-89
referrals 32-33, 84-85
telephone response 86-90
SEE ALSO Client relations, Telephone policies
Encephalomyelitis (equine) 134
Endoscope 127
Equine diseases SEE Diseases, equine
Equine influenza 135, 218-

219
Equine problems SEE Problems, equine
Equine rhinopneumonitis 135, 219
Euthanasia 101-103 SEE ALSO Grief counseling
Eye problems SEE Allergies, Runny eyes

F

Fees
- fee structure 46-49
- price shoppers 46, 114-115
- services/emergencies 54, 90-92 SEE ALSO Client relations, Marketing, Payment policies

Feline diseases SEE Diseases, feline
Feline infectious peritonitis (FIP) 125, 133
Fire 35
Fleas 71, 152-154, 164, 203, 214
Floating 188, 225
Founder 93, 188, 226-227
Fractures 175

G

Gasterophilus 149, 220
Gelding 172, 239
Gestation periods
- canine 206, 257
- equine 222, 257
- feline 207, 257

Gingivitis 179, 213
Grief counseling
- brochures 102-103
- burial arrangements 100, 102
- euthanasia 101-102
- resources 103
- sympathy cards 101

H

Heart failure/heart problems 181, 185, 212-213
Heartworm 125, 144-147, 163, 197-198
Heat cycles 204-207, 222
Hepatitis 131
Home care, instructions for 72-75, 99-100, 172
Hookworm 140, 142
Hospitalized pets 42-43, 96-98 SEE ALSO Client relations
Hyperthyroidism, feline 185

I

Immunizations, SEE Vaccinations 178-182
Infections 183, 213
Influenza, equine SEE Equine influenza
Insect growth regulators/ Insect development inhibitors 153-155

K

Kennel cough 131

L

Lab work
- in-clinic 124-126
- outside 22-23, 126

Leptospirosis 131
Leukemia, feline 125, 133-134, 195
Limping in horses 188
Lyme disease 132, 154, 195, 203

M

Mange, canine
  demodectic (red) 213
  sarcoptic 183, 213
  SEE ALSO Skin problems
Marketing
  brochures 102, 115-116
  exam follow-up 118
  Internet, e-mail 120-121
  lost pets 114
  new clients 114-116
  newsletter 120
  photo albums 119-120
  product education 117
  product follow-up 118
  recall lists 113
  referrals 115-116
  reminder notices 113
  surgery follow-up 113
  waiting room 119-120
  Web sites 121-122
  SEE ALSO Client relations, Telephone policies
Megacolon (massive constipation) 186
Memorial donations 116-117
Microfilariae 144-147

N

Neuter SEE Castration
Nonprescription drugs 158, 164-165

O

OSHA manual 34
Obesity
  canine 182, 204
  equine 188-189
  feline 186, 204
Organization 16-25
Ovariohysterectomy SEE Spay
Oxyuris SEE Pinworm

P

Pain management 171
Parasites, external 152-156
  control of 153-154
  fleas 152-154, 200-203
  ringworm 125, 183-184, 203, 221
  ticks 154-155, 200-203
Parasites, internal 140-150
  bloodworm 147, 187, 220
  bots 149, 220
  canine/feline 140-147
  coccidia 140, 142
  equine 147-150
  heartworm 163, 197-199
  hookworm 140, 142
  pinworm (Oxyuris) 149
  questions about 219-221
  roundworm 141-142, 149
  tapeworm 142-143, 199-200
  whipworm 142-144
Parvovirus 132, 193-195
Payment policies 46-60
  cash 50
  check 50-52
  collection problems 55-60
  credit card 53-54

emergencies 90-92
exceptions 54-60
payment plans 55-60
SEE ALSO Fees
Pinworm (oxyuris) 149
Poison 69, 214
SEE ALSO Emergencies
Policy manual 18-23
Prescriptions SEE Drugs, prescription
Problems, canine 178-184
allergies 183, 213-214
ear problems 180
growths, lumps, tumors 185
mange 126, 183, 213
Problems, equine 187-189
colic 93,149, 187, 221, 226
corneal ulcer 187
dental problems 187-188
diarrhea 221
equine infectious anemia (EIA) 224-225
founder 188, 226
limping 188
obesity 188-189
parasites 147-150
wolf teeth 225
Problems, feline 184-187
abscesses 184
asthma 184
feline urinary syndrome 184-185
growths, lumps, tumors, 185
heart problems 185
hyperthyroidism 185
obesity 186
ringworm 186
Pyometra 174-175

R

Rabies
canine 132
equine 218
feline 134
questions about 192-194
Radiology 126-127
Records
confidentiality 43
payment problems 59
recording calls 41-42
transfer of 32-33
Recall lists 113
Referrals
emergency 30-31, 84-85
marketing 115-116
new client 115-116
Reminder notices 113-114
Rhinopneumonitis, equine 135, 219
Ringworm 125, 203, 221
canine 183
feline 186, 203
Robberies 35
Roundworm 141-142, 149
Runny eyes 181-182, 213

S

Safety 34-35
Salespeople/solicitors 34
Seborrhea 183 SEE ALSO Skin problems
Skin problems
allergies 183, 213-214
mange 126, 183
seborrhea 183

Skin swab 126
Sore throat/tonsillitis 184
Spay (ovariohysterectomy) 171-172, 174-175, 204-205
Sterile conditions SEE Surgery
Strangles 135-136
Supplies, dispensing 164-165
Surgery
  anesthesia 168-171
  castration (neuter) 172-173, 208-209, 223
  cesarean section 174
  common procedures 171-176
  declaw, feline 173, 235
  dewclaw removal 173-174
  ear trim 173
  fractures 175
  home care instructions 72-75, 99-100
  pyometra 174-175
  spay (ovariohysterectomy) 171-172, 204-205
  sterile conditions 169-170
  tail docking 174
  tumors 175

T

Tail docking 174
Tapeworm 142-143, 199-200
Tartar 179
Telephone policies 7-13
  anxious clients 9-13, 97
  doctor's home phone 30
  emergencies 84-90
  follow-up 41-42
  placing callers on hold 8-9
  returning calls 10-13
  SEE ALSO Client relations, Emergencies, Marketing
Tests, diagnostic
  computer-enhanced images 128
  endoscope 127
  importance of 124
  lab tests 124-126
  radiology 126-127
  types of 124-128
  ultrasound 127
Tetanus 136, 219, 253
Ticks 132, 200-203
Tumors 127-128, 175, 181, 185

U

Ultrasonography 127

V

Vaccinations
  canine, types of 130-132
  equine, types of 134-136
  feline, types of 133-134
  importance of 130
  questions about 192-196, 218-219
  scheduling 38-40, 68-69,
  updates 137
Vomiting 92, 132-133, 168, 216, 256

W

Whipworm 142-144
Wolf teeth 225
World Wide Web 121-122
Worms SEE Parasites, internal